Intermittent Fasting For Women Over 50

The Winning Guide To Accelerate Weight Loss, Unlock Your Metabolism And Promote Longevity. It Only Takes A Few Hours Without Food To Detox Your Body!

BONUS: 14-Day Meal Plan & Exercising Routine

By

Sierra Weil

Table of Contents

Introduction

Women over 50 will have a difficult time when it comes to losing weight. Many factors can cause it. The most common cause is a slowed metabolism. The higher your metabolism is, the leaner muscle you have. However, as you age, you lose lean muscle mass and become less involved than you once were.

Intermittent fasting has grown in popularity due to its many health advantages and the fact that it does not limit food choices. According to research, fasting has been shown to increase mental health, metabolism and possibly prevent cancers. It can also protect women over 50 from some nerve, muscle, and joint disorders.

Intermittent fasting limits when and how much you eat for some time. There are several options.

- Every other day, you normally eat during alternate-day fasting. On the days in between, you consume just 25% of the daily calorie requirements in one meal. So, if you eat 1,800 calories on Monday, Wednesday, and Friday, then on Tuesday, Thursday, and Saturday, you'd eat a 450-calorie food (and nothing else).

- In the 5:2 diet, you normally eat for 5 days and then consume only 400 to 500 calories for the next two days.

- Every day is the same with the 16:8 methods: you fast for 16 hours and then eat normally for eight hours, such as between 9 a.m. and 5 p.m.

Intermittent fasting seems to have a wide range of health benefits. The flipping of a metabolic switch may theoretically cause these results.

"Fasting causes glucose (blood sugar) levels to drop. After converting fat into ketones, the body uses fat rather than glucose as a source of energy," Kathy McManus, director of the Department of Nutrition at the Harvard-affiliated Brigham and Women's Hospital, explains. The switch from glucose to ketones as an energy source has a positive impact on body chemistry.

At least in animals, intermittent fasting is linked to a longer lifespan. What is the reason for this? According to recent Harvard research, intermittent fasting can allow each cell's energy-producing engines (mitochondria) to produce energy more efficiently and maintain a more youthful state.

There's also some science at work here, in the form of your body's HGH production. The bodies generate insulin to store glucose from carbs for later use when you eat. You live in a world where most of the meals are regular, and you are constantly bombarded with foods that are high in sugar and fat. It puts you in an anabolic state, which means you're still gaining weight. Food glucose is deposited as fat, resulting in weight gain. Intermittent fasting effectively reverses this mechanism, allowing the cells to use the glucose that has been deposited in the cells for energy. Weight loss occurs as cells reach a catabolic (breaking down) state. HGH is generated in response to your body's need for glucose, but the HGH output is suppressed when you eat because you are getting glucose from outside sources. HGH is a hormone that regulates metabolism and has many benefits for muscle recovery and fat burning. Fasting for short periods has been shown to increase HGH output by up to 5 times.

Reading this book is going to present you with tons of benefits of intermittent fasting. If you like the book, you are welcome to leave a good review.

Chapter No 1: What is Intermittent Fasting?

1.1 What is Intermittent Fasting and Why Should You Practice It?

Intermittent fasting is a method of eating, not a diet. It's a method of planning the foods so that you get the best out of them. Fasting does not alter your eating habits; rather, it changes the timing of your meals.

Why is it important to modify your eating habits?

Most importantly, it's a perfect way to get lean without going on a fad diet or severely restricting your calorie intake. In reality, when you first start intermittent fasting, you'll try to keep the calorie intake constant. (Most people consume larger meals in a shorter period). Intermittent fasting is also a healthy way to maintain muscle mass when losing weight.

The primary motivation for people to pursue intermittent fasting is to lose weight.

Most importantly, since it takes relatively little behavior modification, intermittent fasting is one of the best methods for losing weight while maintaining a healthy weight. It is a positive thing because it means intermittent fasting falls into the category of "easy enough to do, but significant enough to make a difference."

How Does Intermittent Fasting Work?

To comprehend how the intermittent fasting contributes to fat loss, we must first comprehend the fed and fasted states' distinction.

When your body digests and absorbs food, it is in a fed state. The fed condition usually begins when you start eating and lasts 3 to 5 hours as your body digests and absorbs the food you just ate. Since the insulin levels are high while you're in the fed state, it's difficult for the body to burn fat.

During that period, the body enters a condition known as the post absorptive state, which is simply a fancy way of saying that it isn't processing a meal. The post-absorptive condition lasts until you reach the fasted state, which is 8 to 12 hrs after your last meal. Since your insulin levels are poor, it is much easier for your body to burn fat while you fast.

Fasting allows the body to burn fat that was previously unavailable during the fed state.

The bodies are rarely in this fat-burning state because we don't reach the fasted state until 12 hours after the last meal. Many people who begin intermittent fasting lose weight without changing their diet, amount of food consumed, or exercise intensity. Fasting induces a fat-burning state in your body that you seldom achieve on a regular eating schedule.

1.2 Brief Introduction to 16:8 Intermittent Fasting

A common form of fasting is 16:8 intermittent fasting, also known as the 16:8 plan or the 16:8 diet. This plan requires people to fast for sixteen hours/ day and then have all of their calories for the rest of the 8 hours. Fat loss, weight loss, the prevention of type 2 diabetes, and other obesity-related disorders are all suggested advantages of the 16:8 strategy. Please continue reading to know more about the 16:8 fasting plan, which includes how to execute it and disadvantages and health benefits.

What is 16:8 intermittent fasting, and how does it work?

The majority of people who follow a 16:8 intermittent fasting schedule eat their daily calories in the middle of the day. Intermittent fasting, also known as 16:8, is a form of time-restricted fasting. It entails eating for 8 hours and then fasting for the remaining 16 hours of the day. Some people claim that this approach allows the body's circadian rhythm, or internal clock, to function better. The 16:8 diet allows most people to fast at night and for a portion of the morning and evening. They eat the bulk of their calories in the middle of the day. During the 8-hour window, there are no limits on the types or quantities of food consumed. The strategy is relatively simple to execute because of this flexibility.

How to Go About It?

The best way to stick to the 16:8 diet is to choose a 16-hour fasting window that requires sleep time. Some experts recommend finishing your meal in the early evening because your metabolism slows down after that. It is not possible for all. Some people will not be able to eat until 7 p.m. or later in the evening. Even so, it's best to fast for 2–3 hours before going to bed.

People may choose one of the following 8-hour eating windows:

- 9 a.m. to 5 p.m.
- 10 a.m. to 6 p.m.
- Noon to 8 p.m.

People will eat their meals and snacks at their leisure during this period. It's important to eat regularly to prevent blood sugar rises and dips, as well as excessive hunger. Experimenting to find the best eating window and mealtimes for their lifestyle might be necessary for certain people.

Foods to try and advice

While the 16/8 intermittent fasting strategy does not specify which foods to consume and avoid, focusing on limiting or avoiding junk foods is beneficial and healthy. Excessive consumption of unhealthy foods may lead to weight gain and contribute to disease.

- Vegetables and fruits (which can be frozen, fresh, or canned (in water), whole grains, such as oats, brown rice, quinoa, and barley.
- Poultry, beans, fish, tofu, lentils, low-fat cottage cheese, nuts, seeds, and eggs are good sources of lean protein.
- Fatty fish, coconuts, olives, olive oil, nuts, avocados, and seeds are good sources of healthy fats.
- Fiber-rich foods like vegetables, fruits, and whole grains can make a person feel happy and full. Satiety may also be enhanced by eating proteins and healthy fats.

For those adopting the 16/8 intermittent fasting diet, beverages may help with satiety. People sometimes confuse thirst for hunger; drinking water during the day will help you eat fewer calories. During the 16-hour fasting time, the 16/8 diet plan allows you to drink calorie-free beverages like water and unsweetened coffee and tea. It is important to drink fluids regularly.

Tips

People who follow these tips can find it easier to adhere to the 16/8 diet:

- Consuming water frequently during the day, watching less television to minimize exposure to food images may stimulate hunger exercising just before or during the eating window, as exercise may trigger hunger practice mindful eating while consuming meals.
- Practicing meditation during the fasting time to help pass the hunger pangs.
- Cinnamon herbal tea is helpful and can be purchased on the internet.

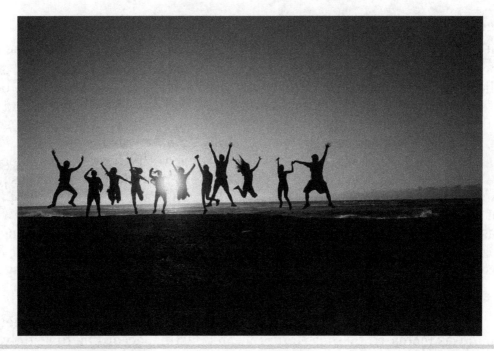

1.3 Advantages of Good Health

Intermittent fasting has been observed for decades by scientists. The results of the research are often inconclusive and inconsistent. However, literature on intermittent fasting, including 16:8, suggests that it could have the following advantages:

Fat loss and weight loss

People who eat for a certain amount of time will help them cut back on their calorie intake. It can also aid in the acceleration of metabolism. According to a 2017 study trusted Source, intermittent fasting causes more fat loss and weight loss in obese women than normal calorie restriction. According to a 2016 study, women who practiced a 16:8 strategy while resistance training for eight weeks saw a reduction in fat mass. Throughout the experiment, the individuals maintained muscle mass.

In comparison, a 2017 study trusted Source reported no difference in weight loss b/w those who practiced intermittent fasting. Alternate-day fasting rather than 16/8 fasting and those who decreased the total calorie intake. Those in the intermittent fasting category have had a high dropout rate.

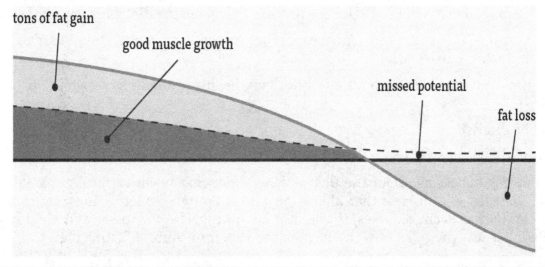

Disease prevention is critical

Intermittent fasting proponents claim that it can avoid a variety of conditions and diseases, including heart disease, type 2 diabetes, diseases in the nervous system and some cancers. However, there is a lack of research in this area. Intermittent fasting appears to be a promising alternative to conventional calorie restriction for type 2 diabetes risk reduction and weight loss in women who are overweight or obese, according to a 2014 study. However, the researchers warn that further research is needed before they can draw definite conclusions. According to a 2018 study, an 8-hour eating window can help adult women with obesity lower blood pressure in addition to weight loss. According to other reports, intermittent fasting decreases fasting glucose by 3–6% in people with prediabetes but has no impact on healthy people. After 4 to 24 weeks of intermittent fasting, it can also lower fasting insulin by 11–57 percent. Fasting for a set amount of time, such as the 16/8 process, can protect learning and memory while also slowing brain disease progression. According to a 2017 annual study, animal studies have shown that this form of fasting lowers the risk of cancer and nonalcoholic fatty liver disease.

Longer life expectancy

Intermittent fasting has been shown in animal research to help animals' live longer lives. Female mice's lifespan was increased by short-term repeated fasting, according to a study. According to the National Institute on Aging, scientists are still baffled as to why fasting can help people live longer lives, despite decades of study. As a result, they are unable to guarantee the practice's long-term protection. There have been few human studies in this field, and the possible benefits of intermittent fasting for human longevity are unknown.

1.4 Risks and Side Effects

Intermittent fasting at a 16/8 ratio has some complications and side effects. As a consequence, the technique isn't suitable for everybody. In the program's beginning stages, potential side effects and threats include hunger, fatigue, and exhaustion. Due to excessive appetite, overeating or consuming unhealthful foods during the 8-hour eating window, you can develop heartburn or reflux. Intermittent fasting should be avoided for people who have a history of disordered eating. Fasting is a risk factor for eating disorders, according to the National Eating Disorders Association. Those with a history of anxiety or depression may also find the 16/8 plan unsuitable. A little research According to Trusted Source, calorie restriction for a short period may help with depression, but prolonged calorie restriction may have the opposite impact. To fully comprehend the implications of these results, further research is needed. Many that are breastfeeding, pregnant, or attempting to conceive can avoid 16/8 intermittent fasting. According to the National Institute on Aging, there is limited evidence to suggest any fasting diet, particularly for adults.

People who want to follow the 16:8 method or other methods of intermittent fasting should first consult their doctor, particularly:

- If they are on medication or have an underlying health problem like low blood pressure or diabetes
- Mental health issues in the past
- A history of eating disorders

Anyone who has questions about the diet or is experiencing negative effects should consult a physician. Diabetes is a disease that affects people. Although evidence suggests that the 16:8 approach can help prevent diabetes, it may not be appropriate for those who already have the disease. People with type 1 diabetes should stop the 16:8 intermittent fasting diet. Under the care of a doctor, some people with prediabetes or type 2 diabetes may try the diet. Before changing their eating habits, people with diabetes who want to follow the 16:8 intermittent fasting method should consult their doctor. Intermittent fasting in the 16:8 ratio is a common method. Weight loss, fat loss, and a decrease in certain diseases' incidence are all possible outcomes. This diet plan could also be easier to stick to than other fasting methods. People who follow the 16:8 intermittent fasting regimen should eat high-fiber whole foods and remain hydrated during the day. The technique is not ideal for all. If you have any doubts or underlying health problems, you should consult a dietitian or a doctor before starting the 16:8 intermittent fasting.

1.5 Best Vitamin D Sources during IF

- yolks of eggs
- oily fish
- Mushrooms
- Foods with extra vitamins
- Obtaining enough vitamin D

Vitamin D is a nutrient produced by the body when a person's skin is exposed to direct sunlight. Vitamin D can also be consumed, although it is not found naturally in many foods. Some varieties of mushrooms and oily fish contain high levels of vitamin D.

The main advantage of vitamin D (according to the Office of Dietary Supplements (ODS)) is that it keeps a person's muscles, bones, and nerves healthy. It also helps in the maintenance of a balanced immune system.

If the chickens that lay the eggs are free-range, they can be contained in the yolks. Vitamin D is also used in some mushrooms.

On the other hand, other plant-based foods do not contain vitamin D. It can be difficult to get enough vitamin D if one's diet is mainly vegetarian or vegan and if one does not or cannot spend much time outside.

If an individual is concerned that they are not getting enough vitamin D from direct sunlight, consuming the foods mentioned below will increase their overall vitamin D levels.

- oily fish
- Swordfish is high in vitamin D and is a good source of it.

Oily fish and fish oils contain some of the highest levels of vitamin D available in food sources.

It may include the following:

- Cod liver oil contains 450 international units (IU) per tsp Trusted Source, 75% of the regularly recommended allowance (RDA).
- Herring: Each fillet of dry-cooked Herring contains 306 IU or 51 percent of a person's RDA.
- Swordfish: Each piece of dry-cooked swordfish contains 706 IU or 117 percent of a person's RDA.

Mushrooms

Specific mushrooms may be a choice if a person doesn't like fish or is vegetarian or vegan. Vitamin D is abundant in some mushroom varieties.

There are some of them:

- Raw maitake mushrooms have 562 IU per 50 grams (g) Trusted Source, 94 % of the recommended daily allowance.

- Dried shiitake mushrooms contain 77 IU per 50 g Trusted Source or about 12% of a person's RDA.

- Mushrooms that have been exposed to ultraviolet (UV) light will contain a lot of vitamin D. This may include the following:

- Raw Portobello mushrooms that have been exposed to UV light produce 568 IU per 50 g Trusted Source, which is 95 percent of a person's RDA.

- Raw white mushrooms that have been exposed to UV light produce 523 IU per 50 g Trusted Source, which is 87 percent of a person's RDA.

Egg yolks

Vitamin D levels in egg yolks can be high, particularly if the chickens are free-range. A dish of scrambled eggs made with two large hen eggs, for example, contains 88 IU Trusted Sources or 15% of a person's RDA.

Fortified foods

Many commonly available foods are high in vitamin D. These foods are fortified with vitamin D or other nutrients.

Extra vitamin D and other nutrients can be found in a variety of foods, including:

- milk from a cow

- the juice of an orange

- Cereals for tea, etc.

Obtaining enough vitamin D

Some cancers and cardiovascular diseases may be resistant to vitamin D.

According to the ODS, people who don't get enough vitamin D in their diet are more likely to have poor bones. A person's bones may hurt, or their muscles may become weak as a result of this. These signs and symptoms can be subtle at first.

Some evidence suggests that vitamin D can play a role in other health benefits, including

- cancer resistance

- hypertension and diabetes

- diseases in the cardiovascular system

- Multiple sclerosis (MS)

However, the ODS claims that there isn't enough proof to know whether this is the situation. Existing research has shown conflicting results.

The RDA for vitamin D is 600 IU for people aged 1 to 70. It is 400 IU for children under the age of one and 800 IU for adults over 70. It implies that an individual receives the bare minimum of direct sunlight.

The common belief is that a person who spends a few hours outside each week will produce enough vitamin D. According to the ODS. However, this can vary significantly depending on:

- The season, the time of day, and whether or not there is cloud cover or smog.
- The color of a person's face, regardless of whether or not they are wearing sunscreen.

Since glass blocks the radiation that produces vitamin D, being in direct sunlight behind a window will not help vitamin D development. It's vital to get enough vitamin D to keep your bones safe. The only way to get enough vitamin D is to spend time outdoors regularly, ensuring that the head, face, and legs are exposed. Consuming enough vitamin D can be difficult, depending on a person's dietary preferences. Vitamin D supplements, which are available for purchase online, could be a good option in this situation. Instead, eat mushrooms, oily fish, and free-range egg yolks if this isn't possible. Are tailored vitamins beneficial to your health?

1.6 Risks and Factors Associated with Supplementing

Companies that market customized vitamins say that their supplements are tailored to a person's unique health needs. Taking supplements in this manner, however, has some drawbacks. The federal government, for example, does not strictly control personalized vitamins. The companies may fail to deliver on their promises, and the vitamins they prescribe may be unsafe.

What exactly are tailored vitamins?

According to some firms, personalized vitamins may be customized to an individual's genetic code, unique health problems, or both.

They're not like conventional dietary supplements, which offer all the same types and quantities of vitamins.

Personalized vitamins are available from a variety of companies in the United States, such as:

- Persona
- Care/of
- Vitl
- Nourished

The majority of those selling customized vitamins say that their customization is based on an online questionnaire that takes just a few minutes to complete. These surveys gather data on a person's level of physical activity, drugs, and health conditions, as well as their consumption of such dietary staples, like calcium-rich foods or vegetables. Companies can also say that their vitamin customization is based on a person's DNA test results. Nutrigenomics Trusted Source is a scientific area that studies how a person's nutrient intake, genetic structure, and health interact. Such businesses claim to predict the likelihood of contracting different diseases based on the test results while also recommending certain vitamins' consumption.

Do they have any health benefits?

There have been several studies on personalized vitamins. There isn't much evidence to back up their advantages, particularly when compared to non-personalized choices. Companies offering personalized supplements are subject to minimal government control in the United States. These vitamins can not only fail to benefit health, but the companies which sell them can also have unreliable or inaccurate health information (according to an older Government Accountability

Office (GAO) report). One of these providers' key arguments is that they customize supplements to a person's specific health requirements. The GAO study investigated this assertion's authenticity by investigating four companies that provide this service using fake profiles. The authors conducted online surveys before submitting DNA samples for processing. The internet sources urged the purchase of costly personalized vitamins after presenting the test results to the study's authors. However, rather than being personalized, the vitamins prescribed for each of the fictional profiles were the same. It is particularly worrying since the profiles were produced using DNA samples from two people with very different lifestyles. Furthermore, according to the American Society of Nutrition (ASN), there is insufficient evidence to suggest that taking multivitamins prevents chronic or long-term diseases in general. Despite limited studies suggesting they can help with some conditions, this is the case.

Risks and factors

Many customized vitamin brands' online surveys and quizzes may not be reliable or accurately interpreted. Nutritional requirements are influenced by a person's medical history and family context. As a result, analyzing online polls and reports is difficult and unlikely to be conclusive or systematic. Because of these variables, a person's doctor is generally the best person to interpret these tests. The American Society of Nutrition warns that consuming vitamins can increase the chances of getting more than the TUI (Tolerable Upper Intake) of some nutrients. It can put your health at risk. For example, if they eat foods fortified with the vitamin, TUI can be exceeded for people who take a folic acid supplement. High folic acid levels can increase the risk of birth defects. Certain forms of cancer, such as prostate cancer, have a trusted source.

Issues arising from an erroneous analysis of DNA tests

When customized vitamin companies provide DNA testing, they're typically looking for things like caffeine metabolism, gluten intolerance, skin antioxidant ability, and other things. They may also be determining the risk of such diseases. According to the Federal Trade Commission (FTC), there is no evidence that DNA tests can be used to customize dietary supplements safely. According to the Federal Trade Commission, it is often difficult to draw definite conclusions regarding health hazards based on DNA samples. A person's chances of contracting a disease are also not exclusively determined by their genes. Rather, it results from a complex relationship between their genes and the foods they eat, their lifestyle, and substances they are exposed to regularly, such as cigarettes or sunlight. The Food and Drug Administration (FDA) Trusted Source warns that misinterpreting DNA tests may lead to two issues. The first is a positive test result for a disease, which does not guarantee that a person will contract it or be serious. A negative result for a specific disease is the second problem. It may simply mean that the test did not look at the precise genetic changes related to the disease. The majority of DNA experiments look at a few genes. As the GAO study concludes, a positive outcome can alarm people unnecessarily and encourage them to spend money on expensive personalized vitamins to stay safe. Furthermore, a negative result could give some people the false sense of being healthy when they are sick.

1.7 Intermittent fasting Has 10 Proven Health Benefits

Intermittent fasting is an eating practice in which you vary between eating and fasting times. Intermittent fasting can be achieved in a variety of ways, such as the 16/8 or 5/2 methods. Numerous studies have shown that it can have important health and cognitive benefits.

Here are ten health benefits of intermittent fasting that have been proven.

1. Alters Gene, Cell, and Hormone Function.

When you don't eat for a while, your body goes through several changes. Your body initiates essential cellular repair processes and adjusts hormone levels to make stored body fat more available. Here are some of the changes that occur during fasting:

- Levels of insulin: Insulin levels in the blood fall significantly, allowing fat to be burned more efficiently.

- Human growth hormone: Growth hormone levels in the blood will rise by up to fivefold. Increased levels of this hormone help with fat loss and muscle growth, among other things.

- Significant cellular repair processes, such as removing waste material from cells, are induced by the body.

- Gene expression: There are beneficial variations in some molecules and genes linked to survival and disease prevention.

These variations in gene expression, hormones, and cell function are linked to several advantages of intermittent fasting. Insulin levels fall, and human growth hormone levels rise when you fast. Your cells also initiate critical cellular repair processes and alter gene expression.

2. Weight loss and belly fat reduction.

Many people who experiment with intermittent fasting do so to lose weight. In general, intermittent fasting allows you to eat fewer meals. You will consume fewer calories unless you compensate by consuming even more during the other meals. Intermittent fasting also improves hormone function, which helps weight loss. Higher growth hormone levels, lower insulin levels, and higher norepinephrine (noradrenaline) levels help the body break down fat and use it for energy. As a result, fasting (short-term) boosts the metabolic rate by 4-14 percent. Intermittent fasting, in other words, operates on both sides of the calorie equation. It increases the metabolic rate while decreasing the quantity of food you consume. According to a study of the scientific literature (2014), intermittent fasting may help in weight loss of about 3-8 percent in 3-24 weeks which is a massive amount. The women also lost 4-7 percent of their waist circumference, suggesting that they lost a lot of belly fat, the disease-causing fat in the abdominal cavity. Intermittent fasting caused less muscle failure than constant calorie restriction. When it is said and done, intermittent fasting may be a very effective weight-loss strategy. More information can be found here: How the Intermittent Fasting Can Help Weight Loss. Intermittent fasting allows you to consume fewer calories while marginally increasing your metabolism. It's a powerful tool for losing weight and belly fat.

3. Lower the risk of Type 2 diabetes by reducing insulin resistance.

In recent decades, type 2 diabetes has become extremely popular. High blood sugar levels in the sense of insulin resistance are the most prominent aspect. Anything that lowers insulin resistance & protects against type 2 diabetes should help lower blood sugar level. Intermittent fasting has been shown to have important benefits for insulin resistance & a significant reduction in blood sugar levels. Intermittent fasting has been shown to lower fasting blood sugar level by 3 to 6 percent & fasting insulin by 20 to 31 percent in human studies. Intermittent fasting also prevented diabetic rats from kidney injury, which is one of the most significant complications of diabetes. It suggests that intermittent fasting could be particularly helpful for people at risk of developing type 2 diabetes.

4. Intermittent fasting can help the body reduce oxidative stress and inflammation.

Oxidative stress is one of the factors that contribute to aging and the development of several chronic diseases. The unstable molecules, known as free radicals, react with and damage other essential molecules such as DNA and protein. Intermittent fasting has been shown in many studies to increase the body's resistance to oxidative stress. Studies show that intermittent fasting may help combat inflammation, which is a major cause of several diseases. Intermittent fasting has been shown in studies to minimize oxidative stress and inflammation in the body. It should help avoid aging and the onset of several diseases.

5. Intermittent fasting may be good for your heart.

Heart disease is currently the world's leading cause of death. Various health indicators (also known as "risk factors") have been related to an increased or decreased risk of heart disease. Intermittent fasting has been shown to improve risk factors, such as total and LDL cholesterol, blood pressure, blood triglycerides, inflammatory markers, and blood sugar levels. However, a large portion of this is focused on animal science. Before any recommendations can be made, further research on humans' heart health effects is needed. Intermittent fasting has been shown in studies to improve cholesterol levels, blood pressure, inflammatory markers and triglycerides, all of which are risk factors for heart disease.

6. Intermittent fasting causes a variety of cellular repair mechanisms.

When we fast, our bodies' cells begin a cellular "waste removal" process known as autophagy. Broken and damaged proteins that accumulate within cells over time are metabolized and broken down by the cells. Increased autophagy has been related to a reduction in the risk of Alzheimer's disease and cancer. Fasting activates the autophagy metabolic pathway, which eliminates waste from cells.

7. Intermittent fasting can help in cancer prevention.

Cancer is a horrific disease that is characterized by uncontrollable cell growth. Fasting has been shown to have a variety of metabolic advantages, including a lower risk of cancer. Intermittent fasting can help prevent cancer, according to promising evidence from animal studies. Human studies are needed. Fasting minimizes multiple side effects of chemotherapy in human cancer patients, according to some evidence. In animal research, intermittent fasting was shown to help prevent cancer. In humans, one study found that it can minimize chemotherapy side effects.

8. Intermittent fasting is beneficial for your mental health.

What is beneficial for the body is frequently often beneficial for the brain. Intermittent fasting increases a variety of metabolic characteristics that are related to brain health. Reduced oxidative stress, inflammation, blood sugar levels, and insulin resistance are all part of this. Intermittent fasting has been shown in experiments on rats to increase new nerve cell development, which could improve brain function. It also raises levels of a brain hormone named brain-derived neurotrophic factor (BDNF), whose lack has been related to depression and other mental illnesses. Intermittent fasting has also been shown to protect against brain damage caused by strokes in animals. Intermittent fasting is beneficial to brain health. It has the potential to promote the development of new neurons while also protecting the brain from injury.

9. Intermittent fasting can reduce the risk of Alzheimer's disease.

The most common neurodegenerative disease in the world is Alzheimer's disease. Since there is no cure for Alzheimer's disease, stopping it from occurring in the first place is important. Intermittent fasting has been shown in rats to postpone Alzheimer's disease or reduce its severity. According to a series of case reports, a lifestyle intervention that included regular short-term fasts substantially boosts Alzheimer's symptoms in 9 out of 10 patients. According to animal studies, fasting may also defend against other neurodegenerative disorders, such as Parkinson's and Huntington's disease. However, further human research is needed. Intermittent fasting may protect against neurodegenerative diseases like Alzheimer's disease, according to animal studies.

10. Intermittent fasting can help you live longer by extending your life span.

One of the most intriguing applications of intermittent fasting is the potential to prolong life span. Intermittent fasting increases lifespan in rats in the same way as constant calorie restriction does. The results of some of these studies were very dramatic. Rats who fasted every other day lived 83 percent longer than rats who didn't. Intermittent fasting has become very common among the anti-aging crowd, although it has yet to be demonstrated in humans. Given the benefits of intermittent fasting for metabolism and a variety of health indicators, it's easy to see how it could help you live a longer and healthier life.

Chapter No 2: The Science behind Intermittent Fasting

2.1 Empirical Data on Intermittent Fasting

Intermittent fasting has been hailed as the key to weight loss, and you've certainly heard the hype. According to leading researcher Satchin Panda, there is scientific evidence for intermittent fasting benefits, neither a guaranteed nor an easy cure. Panda, a circadian biology professor at the Salk Institute for Biological Studies in La Jolla, California, has dedicated his career to researching the human body's complex biochemical processes. Intermittent fasting appears to support human health in many ways, including weight loss, according to his studies in mice and humans. Let's get one thing straight before we get into the science: Intermittent fasting can be achieved in many ways. If you search it, you'll find a slew of alternatives, each with its own set of supporters. The 5:2 diet includes consuming very few calories (approximately 500-600) for 2 days of the week, then eating normally for five days. Alternative-day fasting is another option, which involves consumption of food normally 1 day and then eating none or just 500 calories the next. All intermittent fasting strategies work on the same principle: when your caloric intake is reduced, your body can turn to stored fat for energy. However, intermittent fasting differs from calorie restriction. It can be easier for people to limit calories for short periods than the days, weeks, and months required by traditional diets. Plus, the kind of intermittent fasting Panda studied may have extra advantages. Panda has been focusing on a form of intermittent fasting called time-restricted feeding.

A human consumes all of the calories for a day within an 8-to-12-hour window in this format. Let's pretend you start your day with a cup of coffee at 7 a.m. and end it with popcorn and a soda around 11 p.m. You could turn to consuming breakfast at 8 a.m., including coffee, and finishing your dinner by 6 p.m. if you practice time-restricted eating. You'll be consuming all of your meals within 10 hours, and you'll be skipping desserts, evening snacks, and alcohol calories. But that isn't the whole of the story. Time-restricted feeding seems to be beneficial to the body in more ways than just calorie reduction. Mouse's study from 2012 was the first to say this. They fed the same diet to two genetically identical mice — a lab-mice variant of the regular American diet, high in fat and simple sugar but low in protein.

Although both groups were given the same quantity of food, one group had access to it for 24 hours while the other only had access for 8 hours. Mice are nocturnal animals that sleep during the day and feed at night. When one group of mice was given access to food 24 hours a day, they started eating some of it during the day, when they should have been sleeping.

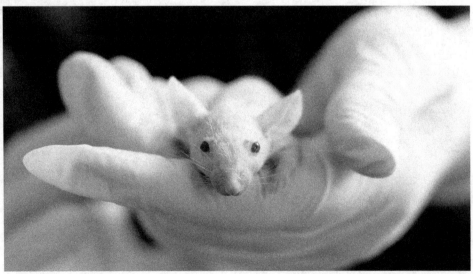

The mice who could feed at any time showed signs of insulin resistance and liver damage after 18 weeks. These conditions did not occur in the mice that ate within an 8-hour window. They also weighed 28% less than mice who had access to food 24 hours a day, even though both groups consumed the same amount of calories a day. Panda recalls, "It was earth-shattering." Until then, he and other researchers believed that weight gain was measured by the total amount of calories consumed rather than when they were consumed.

The experiment was repeated with three different sets of mice, and the findings were the same. The findings were consistent across various types of food and eating windows of up to 15 hours, but the shorter the time, the less weight the mice gained. When the time-restricted mice were given freedom for two days a week, they gained less weight than mice who could eat 24 hours a day.

Scientists then attempted it differently: they moved mice who gained weight due to unlimited feeding to time-restricted feeding. Despite eating the exact number of calories, those mice lost weight and held it off for the duration of the study, which was 12 weeks. They also reduced insulin resistance, which is thought to be related to obesity, though scientists are still confused by the connection. Of course, the human body is more complicated than a mouse's, but these tests were the first example of how crucial timing can be to use food.

According to scientists, many of the human body's mechanisms have been linked to our circadian rhythms in recent years. Most of us are aware that having sunlight first thing in the morning is good for our mood and sleep and that being exposed to light after 9 p.m. from our mobile phones or laptops will disturb our night's sleep. "Similarly, the right food at the right time can nourish everyone, while the wrong food at the wrong time can be junk food. It is processed as fat instead of fuel, making sense when you consider the fundamentals of human metabolism.

Time-restricted eating allows the body to burn fat for longer periods. The bodies use carbohydrates for energy when humans feed, and if you don't use them right away, they are processed as glycogen in the liver or transformed into fat. The bodies run on sugar from the carbs consumed for a few hrs when finished eating for the day before tapping into stored carbs, or glycogen, in the liver. The glycogen in human bodies lasts over several hrs before running out about 8 hrs after you stop feeding, at which point the bodies start to tap into the fat stores.

Humans spend more time in this fat-burning mode of metabolism as they shorten the eating window and prolong the fasting window. However, as soon as they consume food again, even if it's only a coffee cup containing a little milk and sugar, they return to the other technique (storing glycogen and fat and burning carbohydrates). So, if you finish your evening snack at 10 p.m., your body will run out of glycogen and begin burning fat around 6 a.m. If you change your breakfast time from 6 a.m. to 9 a.m., you've given your body 3 extra hours to use fat as fuel.

Panda conducted his time-restricted eating experiments on humans and discovered that they were also promising. In 2015, he and his colleagues attempted to place a small group of people on a 16-week time-restricted eating schedule. Surprisingly, the researchers gave these people no diet recommendations or guidance. Instead, the participants were advised to eat only within a 10- to 12-hour window. They took photographs of their food and texted them to the researchers as they ate. The subjects lost a small amount of weight — an average of just over 8 pounds each — after 16 weeks. According to Panda, they recorded better sleep, more energy in the mornings, and less hunger at bedtime, implying that time-restricted eating has a structural effect all over the body. Although the sample size was too small to draw concrete conclusions, the researchers were pleased that the simple intervention appeared to be simple for participants to adopt and sustain.

Time-restricted feeding has been shown to reduce the risk of diabetes. Panda and his team discovered that after one week of restricting their eating to a nine-hour window, 15 men at risk for type-2 diabetes reported a lower spike in blood sugar after a test meal, indicating increased insulin sensitivity. It can also help in the reduction of cholesterol. Scientists time-restricted the eating of 19 people, the majority of whom were taking medicine to reduce cholesterol, blood pressure, or diabetes. They reduced their overall cholesterol by around 11% on average after 12 weeks of eating within a 10-hour window. Scientists also checked in a year later and learned that roughly 34% of the subjects were only eating willingly in an 8-11 hour window. "It was gratifying that they were able to self-sustain for such a long time," Scientist says. According to some figures, it is good news that 1/3 to 1/2 of dieters regain the extra weight.

According to Scientist, here's how you can practice time-restricted eating. Although some intermittent fasting plans encourage people to drink as much coffee and tea as they like during the day, he advises that you only drink water during the fasting window. It means no coffee, tea, or herbal tea, all of which can alter blood chemistry and are thus forbidden during medical blood tests.

Scientist suggests drinking plain hot water after waking up; it can have a similar soothing effect to coffee. Of course, if you need to be alert in the morning, he says it's fine to have a cup of black coffee —avoid adding creamer, sugar, honey, or other sweeteners. He believes that only one tsp of sugar would be enough to double the blood sugar and turn the body from fat-burning to carb-burning mode.

Scientist suggests that you delay eating breakfast until you've been up for a couple of hours. The hormone cortisol spikes about 45 minutes after people wake up, and high levels of cortisol can impede glucose control. Furthermore, the hormone melatonin, which prepares the bodies for sleep, only lasts two hours after humans wake up. It means that the pancreas, which generates the insulin required to use carbohydrates in the food, is also waking up for the first two hours. Then, two to three hours before bedtime, try to finish the last meal, as this is when melatonin starts to prepare the body, including the pancreas, for sleep.

Although intermittent fasting, in particular time-restricted feeding, has tantalizing promise, it is still early days. Other study groups have backed up some of Scientist's findings since he started his research. People on a time-restricted eating program decreased their calorie consumption despite not being asked to and lost a small amount of weight (according to a report published in Cell Metabolism).

More research into time-restricted eating is needed. There hasn't been any human subject's research that has lasted more than a few months. Fasting's impact on the human body must also be understood, according to experts. The gut microbiome has been shown to shift in mice who limit their eating to an eight-to-nine-hour window, causing them to digest nutrients differently and consume less sugar and fat. Is this something only humans should do? Panda isn't the only one looking into the long-term consequences of time-restricted eating; other studies are starting to examine whether intermittent fasting can protect the brain against neurodegenerative diseases.

Intermittent fasting isn't a magic weight-loss solution. According to some studies, people who follow the 5:2 diet or alternate-day fasting can instinctively eat more before and after their fasting days and reduce their activity on intermittent fasting days, negating the calorie-reducing advantages. Scientist claims that in his studies of time-restricted eating, he's seen some participants gain weight after taking the concept of eating everything they wanted within a window, bingeing on foods they normally avoid. Also, unlike mice, the human body may have mechanisms for slowing metabolism such that you burn fewer calories as you consume less. Finally, whether intermittent fasting is safe for people who aren't trying to lose weight is unknown. In reality, people who suffer from binge-eating disorder or anorexia could be at risk; it's easy to see how trying intermittent fasting could promote these harmful behaviors.

Time-restricted feeding has several benefits over other methods of weight loss: It's easy and simple. Diets are also the luxury of those who can afford them because many people don't have the time or resources to count calories — plan their meals, purchase certain things, and monitor their calories. Anyone who can count time and limit eating and drinking to fixed hours can practice time-restricted eating.

Scientists are currently recruiting 120 people to take part in a time-restricted eating trial. They're also looking at whether firefighters' health can be improved by eating within a 10-hour window. Owing to the frequent disturbance of their circadian cycles, firefighters and other shift workers are more vulnerable to disease.

People who want to lose weight have had to concentrate on modifying their regular menus for a long time. Time-restricted eating can extend the number of variables under our influence.

2.2 Biological Functions on Intermittent Fasting

Intermittent fasting is one of the most common eating plans, which comes as no surprise. You won't have to measure anything or buy any pre-made shakes. Weigh-ins or calorie counting are not needed. All you have to do is stop eating at certain times. It's very easy.

Of course, there are many techniques. The 16:8 diet, in which one fast for 16 hours and instead eats within an eight-hour window, is practiced by most people. There's also the 5:2 diet, in which you cut calories dramatically 2 days a week, and 24-hour fasts, in which you don't eat anything for one day every month.

Significantly restricting when you eat, regardless of the process, can throw the body for a loop and cause a slew of weird side effects. It's possible that intermittent fasting isn't right for everybody. (For example, people with a history of eating disorders should avoid it.)

Before you start a new eating habit, it's important to know what to expect. When you fast intermittently, here's what happens to you mentally, physically, and emotionally.

2.3 IF for Healing the Mind and Body

Intermittent fasting isn't solely recommended for weight loss, according to many health experts. That's because you're not cutting calories or eating less. There are long periods where you are not eating at all. However, many people lose bodyweight because they eat fewer calories when they are not allowed to eat.

It's also less likely that you'll consume a huge meal right before bedtime if you only eat for 8 hrs a day. When you sleep, the metabolism slows down and therefore burns fewer calories. Obesity and diabetes have also been related to nighttime feeding.

Dr. John Morton at Yale Medicine said that intermittent fasting "actually helps prevent you from doing some really bad stuff, including eating a big meal before you go to bed."

You may get extremely hungry. Many people who fast experience hunger pangs, particularly when they first begin. Our bodies are used to using glucose — a sugar obtained from food — as a source of energy during the day. When the body is deprived of food (and therefore glucose), it sends out signals that say, "Hello, aren't you missing anything here?"

When your body becomes accustomed to fasting, it will begin to burn stored body fat rather than glucose for energy. And as you fast for longer periods, your body will become more effective at burning fat for energy.

In short, your appetite should balance, and the hunger pangs are dissipated, according to Morton. Fasters would eventually have fewer cravings and hunger pangs if they fast regularly, he said. Meanwhile, some people might be tempted to overeat due to their hunger. Get enough to eat if your hunger pains are serious enough to interfere with your everyday activities. It's not a smart idea to go hungry. Your moods and energy levels will fluctuate. Fasting has been shown in studies to make certain people feel tired, dizzy, irritable, and depressed. "At first, the energy levels could be poor because you aren't getting the necessary nutrients," said Sharon Zarabi at New York's Lenox Hill Hospital. Your energy levels will return as your body adjusts to intermittent fasting. As your body becomes more effective at using energy, your attitude, mental capacity, and long-term success improve.

There's also some evidence that intermittent fasting can help with depression and anxiety in the long run. When you're hungry or fasting, the body releases a hormone called ghrelin, which has been linked to an elevated mood in high doses.

Your gut health may improve. Intermittent fasting has been shown to enhance gut health in many people. Fasting helps the stomach relax and reboot because it isn't forced to deal with the unpleasant side effects of food, such as gas, diarrhea, and bloating. Whenever you fast, your body is taking a break from trying to metabolize what you just ate. By fasting, humans encourage the gut microbiome to regenerate, which benefits our overall digestive system.

You may be able to reduce the risk of developing chronic diseases. Fasting for short periods has been related to a lower risk of chronic diseases like diabetes and heart disease. It is because fasting decreases inflammation, and reducing inflammation helps the bodies fight chronic inflammatory diseases, including diabetes, heart disease, cancer, and inflammatory bowel disease. Researchers are still trying to find out how and why this occurs, but evidence suggests that when you fast, the body produces less of a type of blood cell called monocytes, known to cause tissue damage and inflammation. It is one of the key reasons why people who fast regularly may live longer and be healthier.

Your heart health will likely improve. Intermittent fasting will help you lower your blood pressure, cholesterol, and triglycerides, which are a form of fat in the blood linked to heart disease if you manage to lose many pounds in the process.

Health experts suggest speaking with a dietitian or physician before starting an intermittent fasting program. There's a major difference between fasting and starvation, and if you don't understand it, you might damage your organs and immune system.

The bottom line is to listen to your body and eat most beneficially.

2.4 Intermittent Fasting Helps Minimize Menopausal Symptoms

Intermittent fasting is one of the most common strategies for losing weight and improving overall health. It means going without food for most of the day and eating all of the meals in a short period.

Intermittent fasting has a long list of benefits, from weight loss to better mental clarity, all of which are backed up by science. This way of eating is ideal for many women, but what about menopausal or premenopausal?

When a woman enters her 40s and 50s, her sex hormones gradually begin to decrease when the ovaries stop processing estrogen and progesterone, which causes menstruation to stop. Menopause is described as a woman not having a period for 12 months in a row, but amenorrhea is far from the only symptom of the change.

Hot flashes, anxiety, vaginal dryness, brain fog, decreased libido, chills, depression, mood changes, night sweats, and an increased risk of heart disease are some of the signs of menopause, which can vary from person to person. There is often a noticeable shift in metabolism for certain women, which usually slows down when estrogen and progesterone levels get out of control, causing weight gain.

Women may become less receptive to insulin during menopause. They may have difficulty processing sugar and refined carbohydrates; this metabolic transition is known as insulin resistance, and it is frequently accompanied by exhaustion and sleeping problems.

Many women find menopause frightening in their lives; they may no longer recognize their bodies, and symptoms like sudden weight gain and brain fog may cause confusion, anxiety, stress, anger, and depression.

Fortunately, women may use intermittent fasting to help them manage the sloping roller coaster of menopause. If you're experiencing fatigue, weight gain, or insulin resistance due to menopause, you may want to give it a shot.

Weight gain is helped by intermittent fasting. Fasting enhances insulin sensitivity, which helps the body absorb sugar and carbohydrates more effectively, reducing the risk of heart disease, diabetes, and other metabolic diseases. Fasting has been shown to reduce depression and stress, boost self-esteem, and promote more positive psychological changes. Fasting has been shown in animal studies to help protect brain cells from stress, clean out waste materials, repair, and improve their performance.

When you have a strategy in place, intermittent fasting isn't all that difficult. Set an eating window that works for you, such as noon to 8 p.m., and make sure you consume all of the calories during that time. It would help if you fasted outside of that window, but you can drink water and non-caloric beverages such as coffee or tea. The 16:8 form of fasting involves fasting for 16 hours a day and eating for just 8 hours a day; it is one of the most basic intermittent fasting processes to follow.

Intermittent fasting is simple and flexible; some people begin with shorter fasting times, such as 14:10 (14 hours of fasting followed by a 10-hour eating window), and gradually increase the fasting time until they achieve the target of 16:8. It would help if you experimented with various fasting plans to see what works best for you because of the ease and flexibility.

Although intermittent fasting is a fantastic tool for most women to help relieve the symptoms of menopause, it is not for all. Those who have a chronic illness or adrenal fatigue may not want to implement an intermittent fasting pattern into their routines.

Many who practice intermittent fasting should pay attention to how they feel during the fasting period; if you become tired, weak, or sick while fasting, it might be better to either shorten the fasting period or stop attempting intermittent fasting altogether. You also don't have to fast every day; you can fast every other day or even a couple of times a week. To prevent complications and ensure that any diet or lifestyle change is correct for you, it's also a good idea to check with a trained and certified medical professional first.

Menopause is a tough time for most women. Still, by making the right dietary and lifestyle adjustments, you can help control the symptoms and remain fit, comfortable, and healthy even when the hormones begin to change things up and finally leave the building.

2.5 Eating Habits When Hitting Menopause

Any risk factors and consequences linked to aging and hormonal shifts are difficult to modify. On the other hand, a healthy diet can help prevent or alleviate such conditions before and after menopause.

Menopause Food Advice

Throughout menstruation, eat a variety of foods to ensure that you get enough vitamins. The following guidelines must be followed because women's calcium and magnesium intakes are often deficient:

Make sure you have quite enough calcium.

Daily, two to four portions of processed foods or calcium-rich items are permissible. Calcium is found in dairy products, bonefish (such as tuna and dried salmon), fruits, and grains. A total of 1,200 mg should be consumed.

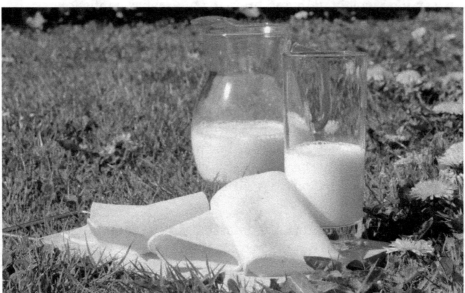

Crank the iron up.

At least three servings of iron-rich foods should be consumed each day. Iron can be found in lean red meat, livestock, pork, chickens, green leafy vegetables, nuts, and fortified grain products. For older people, the recommended daily iron intake is eight milligrams.

Make sure you have enough fiber.

High-fiber foods, such as whole-wheat bread, cereals, pasta, rice, and fresh fruits and vegetables, will help you feel better. Many grown women should be given about 21 grams of fiber per day.

Eat fruit and veggies.

Consume at least 1 1/2 cup of fruit and 1/2 cup of vegetables every day.

Pay heed to the marks.

The information in the product description will help in making the best choices for a healthy lifestyle.

Make sure to drink lots of water.

As primary care, drink 8 cups of water a day. It is sufficient for the healthiest people daily.

Keep a stable weight.

If you're overweight, cut down on serving sizes and eat fewer high-fat meals. Don't skip meals, however. It would be beneficial if you were supported by a professional nutritionist or a doctor to work on your ideal body weight.

Reduce the diet of large foods.

Fat can account for no more than 25 to 35 percent of total calorie intake. Limit processed foods to less than 7% of total caloric intake per day. Sugar that has been refined boosts fat storage and raises the risk of a heart attack. It can be found in milk, processed foods, ice cream, and butter. Limiting the amount of cholesterol consumed each day to 300 mg or less. Trans fats should be avoided, used in vegetable oils, baked goods, and some margarine. As a result, trans-fat raises cholesterol, increasing the risk of heart disease.

Using salt and sugar in moderation.

High cholesterol is linked to a diet high in salt. Avoid fried, sodium-rich, and barbecued meats since they contain high levels of cancer-causing nitrates.

Limit your alcohol consumption to one or two drinks a day.

Foods that may assist with menopausal symptoms.

Flavonoids (plant estrogenic effects) function as a weak hormone source in the brain's soil food sites. For this purpose, soy can help to alleviate the effects of menstruation, but research findings are mixed. Some can help with cholesterol reduction and are also used to treat menopausal symptoms and mood changes. Isoflavones should be used in items like yogurt and oat milk.

What Foods Do You Need To Stop Through Menopause?

Avoiding certain foods and drinks like fried foods, coffee, and alcohol during menopause will help you avoid menopausal symptoms.

Vitamins intake during menopause

Since there is a direct link between the absence of hormones after menstruation and the development of osteoarthritis, the supplements mentioned below, when combined with a healthy diet, may help delay the onset of this disorder:

Calcium is a vital nutrient. If you think you could benefit from a calcium supplement, consult your doctor first. According to a 2012 study, taking prenatal vitamins in only some people can increase the risk of heart attacks. Growing calcium from food sources in the diet did not increase the risk, according to the report.

Folic acid allows calcium to be absorbed by the skin. Every day, people between the ages of 51 and 70 could get 600 IU. Those over the age of 70 can receive 800 IU per day. Taking more than 4,000 IU of vitamin D per day is not recommended because it can damage the kidneys and weaken the bones.

How to Drop Pounds through Menopause?

It may seem impossible to lose weight before or after menopause.

Hormonal changes, depression, and the effects of aging will all work against you.

However, you can do a few things to make losing weight more convenient during this period.

Why is it that menstruation makes losing weight so difficult?

A woman is actually in menopause if she hasn't had her period in 12 months. At this stage, losing weight would be difficult for her. Many women find that they gain weight quickly as their hormones shift. Excess weight during menstruation is caused by a variety of causes, including:

Hormone fluctuations: High and very low testosterone levels can lead to an increase in fat storage.

Muscle mass loss: This is attributed to age, hormonal shifts, and a sedentary lifestyle.

Insufficient sleep: Many women fail to sleep after menopause, and sleep loss has been related to excess weight.

Increased insulin resistance: Women develop insulin resistance as they age, making weight loss more difficult.

Furthermore, fat deposition shifts from the buttocks and waist to the belly during menopause. Cardiac failure, myocardial infarction, and diabetes are also increased risks.

As a result, strategies for reducing belly fat are particularly important at this stage in a woman's life. While calorie intake is essential, diets that are close to zero are ineffective in the long run. To be balanced, you must have a caloric deficit. During and after menopause, a woman's resting resources, or the number of calories she burns at rest, decreases. While it can seem appealing to attempt a crash diet to lose weight quickly, this is the most difficult thing anyone can do. Calorie restriction causes muscle fatigue and lowers carbohydrate intake, according to a report. While very-low-calorie diets can help you lose weight quickly, their effects on muscle strength and mitochondrial rate make it difficult to keep the weight off. Besides, bone loss may occur due to insufficient food intake and a reduction in muscle mass. It puts you at a high risk of breaking a bone.

According to a report, "dietary moderation," such as regulating portion sizes rather than drastically reducing calories, can also help people lose weight. Maintaining your metabolic performance and increasing the amount of exercise you lose as you age. It can be achieved by adopting a long-term healthy lifestyle.

Synopsis

A calorie surplus is needed to lose weight. On the other hand, taking such drastic corrective steps causes excess weight loss, hastening the aging oxygen consumption decline.

Diets for menopause that are both safe and successful

The Eating Low-Carb

Low-carb diets are effective for weight loss and can reduce belly fat in a variety of studies.

Although peri- and menopausal women are included in some low-carb trials, only a few further studies have focused on this group.

In one study, postmenopausal women who followed a low-carb diet for six months lost 21 pounds (9.5 kg), 7% of their body weight, and 3.7 inches (9.4 cm) off their waist.

Furthermore, carbohydrate intake does not have to be too low to result in weight loss.

Another study found that a paleo diet of about 30% carbohydrate calories resulted in greater excess fat and weight reduction after two years than a reduced diet.

Here's where you can learn more about the restricted diet. It includes a menu and a meal plan.

The Cuisine of the Atlantic

Although the Mediterranean Diet is well-known for encouraging health and lowering the risk of heart disease, studies show that it can also help people lose weight. Like reduced diet research, most Aegean diet experiments have focused on both sexes rather than just a long way in supporting or premenopausal women. In one group of women and men aged 55 and up, those who followed a Vegan diet saw significant abdominal fat reductions. Learn this for a balanced eating plan that includes a menu and a meal schedule.

A Vegan or Sustainable Diet

Vegetarian diets have also been shown to help people lose weight. One study of postmenopausal women found that those who followed a vegan diet lost weight and improved their health. However, a more versatile vegetarian approach involving milk and eggs has been shown to work well in older women.

2.6 The Safest Weight Reduction Styles of Fitness

People get less interested as they get older. Exercise, on the other hand, can be essential than ever during or after menopause. It will improve your mood, aid weight loss, and protect your bones and muscles. Weight or band strength training will help you keep or even gain lean muscle mass, which normally decreases with hormonal changes or as you get older. Although all types of resistance training are beneficial, recent research suggests that doing more repetitions is better, particularly in reducing belly fat.

Aerobic exercise (muscles of the lungs) is also beneficial to postmenopausal women. Studies show that you can lose weight and keep your muscle mass while doing so. A combination of weight physical fitness exercises could be the best way.

Synopsis

Resistance and isometric exercise can promote fat loss also preventing the loss of muscle that occurs during menopause.

Weight Reduction Hints through Menopause

Here are many strategies to boost the quality of life through menopause.

Get a Full Night's Sleep

To maintain a healthy weight, you must get enough sleep. People who sleep less have higher ghrelin levels, the hunger hormone, lower insulin, the fullness hormone, and are more likely to become obese. Many menopausal women have difficulty sleeping, leading to cramps, night sweats, stress, and other physical symptoms of hormone deficiency.

Homeopathy and Talk therapy

Women with low oestrogen symptoms can benefit from cognitive therapy, a psychological condition used to treat depression. However, no trials involving menopausal women have been conducted.

Chiropractic treatment may also be beneficial. In one study, it reduced nausea by a median of 33%. An analysis of multiple studies found that acupuncture can help with symptoms and sleep by raising testosterone levels.

Consider a Stress-Relieving Process

Tension management is also necessary during the hormonal phase. Stress causes high cortisol levels linked to belly fat and increases the risk of heart failure. Yoga also help children in relieving anxiety and pain. When given in 100 mg doses, Pycnogonid has been shown to relieve depression and menstrual cramps.

Other Ideas for weight reduction that function

There are a few more weight-loss options for people of all ages, whether or not they are menstruating.

- Eat a well-balanced diet. Protein makes you feel full and satisfied, increases your metabolic rate, and helps you lose weight when you eat healthily.

- Milk is present in the food. Milk products, according to studies, will help you lose fat while maintaining muscle mass.

- Consume a variety of fiber-rich foods. Flaxseeds, Brussels sprouts, avocados, and vegetables are examples of moderate foods that can help with weight loss by boosting insulin response, suppressing appetite, and suppressing appetite.

- The coffee and Eugenol in Earl Grey can help you eat carbs, particularly when combined with resistance training.

- Make mindful eating a habit. By reducing stress and enhancing your relationship with food, mindful eating will help you eat less.

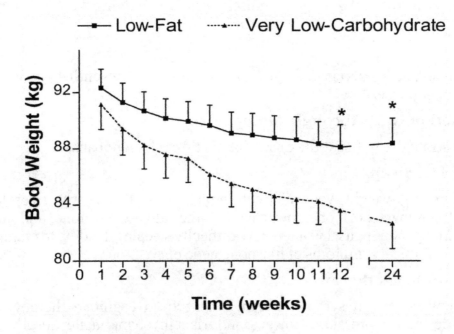

2.7 Intermittent Fasting, Autophagy, and Longevity

Another element of intermittent fasting that is interesting and ground-breaking is its anti-aging impact and the benefits it brings to longevity. It is mainly accomplished by autophagy, which is your body's normal way of eliminating damaged cells then replacing them with new, healthier ones. It's similar to recycling. It is very exciting in terms of long-term sustainability. It is a safe, natural way to replace old cells and turn back the clock to develop new ones. Autophagy is a natural process that our ancestors instilled in us to provide nutrition to the body (self-eating). Of course, this won't last forever, but because you'll be eating every day, your body won't be able to sustain it. When the cells become stressed, intermittent fasting increases autophagy. Autophagy is activated to protect and replenish the body. It prolongs lives. A doctor tested all of these ideas on rats. What he's discovered is incredible. He was able to demonstrate unequivocally that CR would extend the lifetime of rats by 30%. There are no medications or medicines involved, only a common trick that we can all use.

Chapter No 3: The Protocols of Intermittent Fasting

Although some research has shown the benefits of intermittent fasting, such as weight loss, lower blood pressure, and improved metabolic health, further research is required, especially on the long-term effects of intermittent fasting. There's also the question of long-term sustainability. It is not for all to seriously limit calories or go without food for long periods. According to some studies, those who follow intermittent fasting are less likely to stick to it than those who attempt to lose weight on more natural foods. Fasting is a good way to lose weight, but so have other methods like maintaining a well-balanced diet and exercising. According to one study, fasting is no more effective than other well-balanced weight loss methods or blood sugar control. While some people may find IF to be sustainable, others may find that this solution isn't for them. When you start IF, it is recommended that you first figure out how you'll integrate this eating style into your daily life, particularly when it comes to social activities and staying busy. There are different types of intermittent fasting as briefly described below.

1. Alternate day fasting

Every other day, you'll do an "updated" easy. For example, on fasting days, keep your calorie intake to 500 calories, or around 25% of your regular intake. Return to your usual, balanced diet on nonfasting days. (There are strict exceptions to this method, such as eating calories on alternating days rather than 500.)

One study found that people who followed this IF trend for 6 months had significantly higher LDL (or bad) cholesterol levels six months after quitting the diet.

2. Time-restricted eating (example: 16/8 or 14/10 method)

You can set fasting and eating windows in this option; you fast for 16 hours a day and only eat for eight. This method is popular because most people already fast while sleeping. It's realistic because it helps you stretch your overnight fast by missing breakfast and not eating until lunchtime.

3. The twice-a-week method – 5:2

This form of IF focuses on restricting your calories to 500 a day for 2 days a week. You eat a balanced and regular diet for the other 5 days of the week.

This plan typically involves a 200-calorie meal and a 300-calorie meal on fasting days. When fasting, it's important to concentrate on high-fiber and high-protein foods to help fill you up while keeping calories down.

You can fast on any two days (for example, Tuesdays and Thursdays) as long as there is a nonfasting day in between. On nonfasting days, make sure you consume the same amount of food as you usually would.

4. Overnight Fasting

This method is the most simple of the bunch, and it involves fasting for 12 hours every day. Consider the following scenario: Choose to avoid eating by 7 p.m. after dinner and start eating at 7 a.m. the next morning with breakfast. At the 12-hour mark, autophagy still occurs, but the cellular benefits are milder, according to Shemek. It is the bare minimum of fasting hours she advises.

This approach has the advantage of being simple to implement. You still don't have to miss meals; what you're doing is cutting out a bedtime snack (if you ate 1, to begin with). However, this approach does not fully benefit from the advantages of fasting. If you're fasting to lose weight, a smaller fasting window ensures you'll have more time to eat, which does not help you consume fewer calories.

5. Eat Stop Eat

This strategy differs from others in that it emphasizes flexibility. Fasting is simply abstaining from food for a while. You agree to a resistance training regimen and one or two twenty-four-hour fasts per week. "When the fast is done, eat responsibly and act as though it never happened.

Eating wisely means returning to a regular eating routine in which you don't binge because you've just fasted, but you still don't starve yourself or consume less than you require. Fat loss is best achieved by combining intermittent fasting with routine weight training, according to Pilon. You will consume a significantly higher number of calories on the other 5 or 6 nonfasting days if you go on one or two twenty-four-hour fasts throughout the week. He claims that this makes it simpler and more fun to finish the week in a calorie deficit without feeling forced to go on a strict diet.

6. Fasting for the whole day

You only eat once a day here. According to Shemek, some people prefer to eat dinner but then not consume until the next day's dinner. That means you'll be fasting for 24 hours. It is not the same as the 5:2 form. Fasting times are usually 24 hours (lunch to lunch or dinner to dinner), while 5:2 requires a 36-hour fast. (For example, you could eat dinner on Sunday, then go on a 500-600 calorie fast on Monday before breaking it with breakfast on Tuesday).

The benefit is that, if done for losing weight, eating an entire day's worth of calories in 1 sitting is extremely difficult (though not impossible). This approach's disadvantage is that it's difficult to get all of the body's nutrients with only one meal. Not to mention, sticking to this strategy is difficult. By the time dinner arrives, you may be hungry, leading you to consume less-than-healthy, calorie-dense foods. Consider this: When you're hungry, broccoli isn't exactly the first thing that comes to mind. According to Shemek, many people drink too much coffee to satisfy their appetite, disturbing their sleep. If you don't eat, you can experience brain fog during the day.

7. Pick-Your-Own-Day Fasting

It's more like a pick-your-own adventure. According to Shemek, you can do time-restricted fasting every other day or once, maybe twice a week (fast for 16 hours, eat for 8). That means you could have a regular day of eating on Sunday and quit eating by 8 p.m., start eating again at noon on Monday. It's the equivalent of missing breakfast a few times a week.

What are some of the most popular methods?

- Method 16/8: Just eat from 11 a.m. to 7 p.m. or from noon to 8 p.m.
- The 14/10 method: only consuming between the hours of 10 a.m. and 8 p.m.

This method can be performed as much as you'd like, or even once or twice a week, depending on your preferences.

It may take a few days to find out the right eating and fasting windows for this process, particularly if you're very active or if you wake up hungry for breakfast.

Fasting is a popular diet trend that has recently gained popularity.

Fasting may be done in various ways, each with its own set of differences – most notably in fasting/feeding times.

What is intermittent fasting?

Intermittent fasting involves a single daily "eating window" of 4-8 hours.

What is every other day fasting?

You wouldn't consume after every other day of normal eating, or after every two days of normal eating, if you practice alternate-day fasting.

Each strategy is based on the central tenet of lowering total calorie consumption to lose weight.

Is one form superior to the other? Is fasting better than calorie restriction daily? Should one fast and exercise at the same time? Is it permissible for someone to eat or drink something during the fast, like coffee?

3.1 Alternate-Day Fasting

ALTERNATE-DAY FASTING

DAY 1	DAY 2	DAY 3	DAY 4	DAY 5	DAY 6	DAY 7
Eats normally	24-hour fast OR Eat only a few hundred calories	Eats normally	24-hour fast OR Eat only a few hundred calories	Eats normally	24-hour fast OR Eat only a few hundred calories	Eats normally

To begin, consider how many of your days go and determine when the best times not to eat are. We want to eat all the time in the United States, but don't worry about what you want to eat – think about when you don't want to eat. The majority of people miss breakfast in favor of eating in the early or late afternoon. However, if you wake up hungry, there is no hard and fast rule to eat breakfast. If you want to feast yourself before bed, that's also an option.

Since most people aren't especially hungry in the morning and can get through the first few hours fairly quickly, they don't want to be hungry when going to sleep, so the feeding cycle ends a few hours before sleep. To begin, pick a few days during the week to "test" it out. Then head into the 2nd week with a well-thought-out strategy. Using a broader feeding window, such as 8 hours, for at least the first few days. Since you are still sleeping for 8 hours, you are just fasting for about half of the day. Work your way down from 7 hours to 6 hours, 5 hours, 4 hours, and eventually 3 hours.

Some people prefer to stick to an 8-hour eating window, which can be efficient. When most people mention it, they refer to it as a 24:1 ratio, such as 16:8 for sixteen-hour fasts or 20:4 for twenty-hour fasts. You can consume "as much as you want" during eating time, but this is not a scientific reality. If you consume 10,000 calories of ice cream in four hours, you will most likely gain weight. However, eating eight and a half containers of Ben & Jerry's in four hours (one container every 30 minutes) is not something you want to do.

One of the forms that IF works is by decreasing the total amount of food consumption.

Since you can only consume so much before being full and losing the ability to eat, your overall weekly calorie intake would be decreased. Unlike traditional diets, which require a modest calorie reduction for a day and leave you feeling hungry all day, intermittent fasting maintains you stuffed for a few hours each day. Many people find that sticking to the feeding windows increases compliance, while "grazing" on a moderate, consistent calorie-restricted diet destroys the diet.

Planning for intermittent fasting

Alternate day fasting is close to intermittent fasting; however, you just fast 3-4 days a week instead of fasting every day. Hold on – don't get too excited just yet! Fasting days are a bit more serious, and you can't eat as much as you like on regular days. Fasting on alternate days is just what it sounds like. You fast on alternate days, so before you begin, think about which days will be best for fasting. Don't choose Friday if your office has bagel Fridays and you want bagels. If you and your family like going out to eat on Saturdays, avoid them. Choose Wednesday if your mother-in-law's cooking is bad and she still hosts large family dinners on Wednesday. Fasting days aren't necessarily full fasts. They can be one-meal days with very low-calorie intake.

On fasting days, calories are consumed in the range of 0 to 800 for the whole day. Go ahead and eat the meal to get some nutrition and satiety early on in the process.

When you've gotten used to fasting, try it for an entire day! You might find it liberating not to have to think about the food at all during the day. Similarly, if you aren't thinking about that one special meal, your mind is free to think about other, more enjoyable or productive things.

Consume a regular amount of food on nonfasting days. On an intermittent fasting diet, don't go crazy and overeat like a twenty-four-hour eating window. You can't do much damage in four hours, but trying to eat anything at a 24-hour all-you-can-eat buffet would certainly negate any benefits of the fast.

On an intermittent fasting diet or alternate-day fasting diet, what types of food should be eaten?

Eat whatever you want! However, the approach is far from ideal from a clinical and scientific perspective. Whatever dietary plan or nutritional approach you adopted before implementing specific diet practices, such as fasting (or the opposite – eating every 3-4 hours or 6 small meals a day), you'll probably want to keep eating certain foods during your alternate-day fasting diet or intermittent fasting. Making so many major changes at once is difficult. That isn't to say you can't; if you believe you can, go for it. When we think about what's best, we'll think about something high in protein. The issue of whether to eat high-carb or low-carb remains debatable, and it may even be moot if you're fasting, but you can use either method.

Intermittent fasting and protein

Let's talk about protein for a moment. You can consume at least 1.2 grams of protein per kilogram of body weight per day before it becomes difficult – which it won't unless you're fasting all day. Total calorie consumption is the most important factor in weight loss; protein is the second factor. Rich protein diets, particularly when combined with caloric restriction, yield better muscle retention and more fat loss than low protein diets. Protein, on the other hand, cannot be over-consumed!

Adding 800 calories of protein to your daily calorie intake does not increase body weight or fat. Intermittent fasting causes you to eat a low-protein diet, you will most likely lose weight, but you will also be unhappy with your looks.

What is the reason for this? You keep the same fat-to-muscle ratio if you lose muscle tissue at the same rate as fat tissue. As a result, you'll still have the same proportion of fat on top of your muscles and appear fat – slim fat if your body weight is natural. Consider the much-desired abs. You can't see your abs if fat is covering them, and you don't look healthy. Similarly, if you don't have any abs, to begin with, you'll get the same result. Even if you don't want to gain muscle, protein is needed to keep the muscle you already have!

There's a common concern about eating during a fast that's linked to this. What can you eat during a fast? You're not supposed to drink anything but water, according to the rules. Black coffee, BCAA/EAA supplements, and MCT/coconut oil or ketone supplements are a few items that people are lenient on.

Amino acids

Amino acid supplements contain calories, but supplement companies aren't allowed to mention them on supplement facts panels since they aren't intact protein. They have the same number of calories per gram as protein, which is four. They technically do break a fast, but the difference in terms of weight loss is negligible. It could be less negligible for other health or longevity advantages.

Coffee

MCT oil, coffee, and ketones are all calorie-dense foods. With just 10 calories in a cup of black coffee, it's a negligible addition to every diet (coffee improves long-term health).

Ketones and MCTs

By increasing ketones in the blood, MCTs/ketones "induce fasting," however, this is artificial fasting. It is to say that having coffee, MCT, ketones, or BCAA once during the fast isn't a big deal. Black coffee can be drunk freely as the caffeine consumption rate increase will offset the coffee's calories.

Diet drinks

While some artificial sweeteners may trigger an insulin or glucose spike, this is a minor side effect. They are saccharin, sucralose, and aspartame. Some sugar alcohols, especially maltitol and sorbitol, have the same impact.

Then there's this question that always seems to come up when it comes to fasting...

Do one try the keto diet?

Fasting is better in ketosis. Let's face it: there's no way around it. No, you don't need to eat a ketogenic diet on eating days/windows because you'll most likely reach ketosis just by fasting.

If your only aim is to lose weight and stick to your fasting diet, keto-adaptation will make fasting cycles seem more manageable because the body is already willing and able to use fat as fuel. As a result, the feelings of "OMG, I'm starving" are less frequent and come on more slowly. Eating proteins and fats instead of carbohydrates increases satiety on its own, which can enable you to consume less without your understanding – known as auto regulation. You eat less if you get full faster.

Is fasting a bad idea if you're an athlete?

The simple answer is yes, but this isn't always the case. Fasting will potentially improve athletic performance if done correctly. Of course, if you're fasting before a race or competition, you'll feel awful. Depending on the type of exercise and various other factors, fasting for a while after or before a training session can improve exercise adaptations. Fasting before a workout makes the workout more complicated, according to one simplified concept.

If there's one thing we know about training, it has to be challenging to be successful (there are exceptions, but generally speaking). If you don't have enough energy (calories) to complete the workout, it will certainly become more difficult to train. Fasting can boost some adaptations such as mitochondrial biogenesis, fat loss, and efficiency, but it also limits your total exercise volume and intensity.

In general, you keep the balance by doing high-intensity work (sprints, some weight training) while eating and lower-intensity work (cycling, general running, aerobic, or weight lifting etc.) while fasting.

It is similar to the idea of carbohydrate periodization discussed in one of our other papers; however, it is more of a carbohydrate quick than a complete fast in this case. It is a valid technique that you can incorporate into a competitive season or save for the offseason.

These types of items are less important if you're an involved yet non-competitive person. It would help if you still exercised, so there's no need to be concerned with your workouts' timing about your meals.

Fasting diets, like any other diet, are much more effective when combined with an exercise regimen. Caps lock is needed – there is a major difference. If you want to be at your best, don't forget about resistance training!

If you're somewhere between a casual exerciser and a professional athlete, it's worth your time to try and time your workouts and fasting correctly.

In other words, if exercise is one of your top three lifestyle goals, follow the general guidelines outlined above. You'll be frustrated if your runs become more difficult or if you can't complete as many reps as you once did.

Fasting tips for alternating days

Fasting reduces overall calorie consumption, which helps with weight loss and fat loss. That's right, and it's the same as normal dieting. Are you dissatisfied? Don't be that way! There are a couple of other topics to discuss here. The key role is calorie reduction. When total calorie intake is regulated in a laboratory environment, fasting is almost identical to regular dieting for weight loss.

Similarly, in proportion to the degree of calorie restriction, alternate day fasting and intermittent fasting are equally efficient. There are, however, a few advantages of fasting. Control is one of them.

Fasting aids in the development of self-control in dieters and decreases the need to overeat. If you've ever followed a traditional diet, you know that what you're supposed to eat is never enough, and you still want to eat more. Intermittent fasting or alternate-day fasting, on the other hand, causes you to be hungry for some time, then full, then again hungry, then again full.

It's easier to keep your sanity if you "teach your body" that it's okay to be hungry for a while because the food will arrive soon. It isn't the technical way it works, but it's what you'll most definitely see and experience. In terms of the scientific aspects... Fasting can help with glucose and insulin balance. The fasting duration, as well as its repetition over time, "teaches the body" to regulate blood glucose levels better. While this is just a slim relation to body weight, it has greater implications for overall health and longevity. It may be due to mild ketosis and the ability to burn ketones and fats for energy. There is little need to "fat-adapt" in a metabolism (glucose-dominated), such as a high or regular carb diet with steady yet less-calorie intake.

When body fat is the only energy source, mitochondrial biogenesis, mitochondrial health, circadian rhythm, sirtuin activation, cyclic AMP activity, respiratory chain function, inflammation status, and other fascinating mechanisms improve, eventually leading to increased longevity.

It is one of the reasons why some people think it's safe to eat ketones or MCTs.

It is probably not a big deal, but if you're trying to fast, don't eat them – just let your natural ketone development take care of itself; it will happen even if you eat carbs during the feeding cycles (starvation ketosis vs. nutritional ketosis).

Fasting has its own set of potential benefits for athletes, especially endurance athletes.

It may be attributed entirely to the loss of body fat (which was 11 percent higher in the fasting group), but one study showed that fasting increased the exercise economy significantly.

This improved economy occurred at various intensities, ranging from 50 percent VO2Max to 70 percent VO2Max and the threshold. After the fasting period, energy consumption during exercise was reduced by over 10%, and over 7 beats per minute decreased heart rate. It was followed by a drop in blood lactate levels as well as athletes' expectations of exertion. Take this with a grain of salt since this study had a calorie limit of over 30% but no control group.

Other than weight loss and probably increased stamina, we don't know any advantages for other athletes. However, as with "normal" calorie restriction, this can come at the expense of muscle mass loss.

BCAA can be supplemented during a fast to improve anabolic signaling and counter the extremely up-regulated catabolic signals caused by fasting. Without adding many calories, this will help retain more muscle, which would help in the long run.

Is it a diet or just plain "not eating"?

Fasting is generally not harmful. It's not that complicated if you take it slowly at first. One of the few disadvantages of fasting is avoiding food during the day, but it becomes part of the routine after a while.

The only other downside is the possibility of risking lean muscle tissue development. When your energy level is low, your body may not form new muscle tissue and may even break down existing muscle tissue. It isn't a huge deal for the vast majority of endurance athletes. However, for many people, the benefits far outweigh the disadvantages.

Fasting is more fun than traditional dieting, considering how difficult it can seem if you've never done it. One of the most common problems with weight loss diets is that most people give up too soon or cheat too much to be productive. It is easier to achieve success when there are specified criteria and basic rules for fasting. Furthermore, prolonged fasting cycles can have some long-term health and lifespan benefits. Performance can be changed for certain individuals under the right conditions. If you've been debating whether or not to give it a try, it's probably best to just do it!

3.2 16:8 Fasting

The 16:8 diet is a form of time-restricted fasting that can help you lose weight or improve your health. On the 16:8 diet, you drink only unsweetened drinks such as water, coffee, and tea for 16 hours per day. You can consume all of your meals and snacks during the remaining eight-hour window. The majority of people do this by fasting overnight, missing breakfast, and taking the first meal in the afternoon. There are no foods that are inherently forbidden during that period, but some people can adhere to the keto diet at mealtimes to speed up their weight loss. Although the word intermittent fasting (or IF) might be unfamiliar to many, the practice isn't dissimilar to how the ancestors lived: During the day, hunt, gather, and eat; during the night, sleep and fast.

THE 16:8 DIET

	DAY 1	DAY 2	DAY 3	DAY 4	DAY 5	DAY 6	DAY 7
MIDNIGHT							
4 AM	FAST	FAST	FAST	FAST	FAST	FAST	FAST
8 AM							
12 PM	First meal	First meal	First meal	First meal	First meal	First meal	First meal
4 PM	Last meal by 8PM	Last meal by 8PM	Last meal by 8PM	Last meal by 8PM	Last meal by 8PM	Last meal by 8PM	Last meal by 8PM
8 PM	FAST	FAST	FAST	FAST	FAST	FAST	FAST
MIDNIGHT							

Is 16:8 fasting good for weight loss?

According to some reports, there is practically no difference between people who practice intermittent fasting daily and those who merely reduce their total calorie intake.

A growing body of evidence suggests that improving the nutritional quality of what you already consume (fruit, veggies, whole grains, lean protein, and healthy fats) is a better approach than fasting or calorie counting. Furthermore, evidence indicates that any possible advantages from fasting are easily undone during the cycle's eating process, as appetite-suppressing hormones turn gears, making you feel even hungrier than you did before.

However, some dieters who struggle to stick to the restrictive diet or the prescribed meal plans can benefit from regular fasting; pilot study (in 2018) indicates that a 16 by 8 fasting program may help the obese dieters to lose weight even without counting every calorie they consume. This method of fasting can also help people who are struggling with other weight-related problems, such as high blood pressure. According to a new scholarly review, a 16/8 fasting plan can help the body improve blood sugar control naturally while lowering blood pressure.

Is it healthy to fast for 16 hours a day?

16:8 diets, for example, is based on the idea that fasting decreases oxidative stress in body, which may reduce inflammation and the risk of chronic diseases.

According to new study published in Cell Metabolism, fasting gives the metabolic functions, absorptive and digestive hormones, and vital organs a break. Fasting has been related to reducing insulin resistance's susceptibility over time because the bodies secrete insulin to help the cells consume sugar. (Having elevated insulin levels is a risk for many diseases).

On the other hand, fasting had been related to an increase in LDL cholesterol in studies (the "bad" kind). Intermittent fasting may cause nausea and dizziness, as well as low blood sugar and dehydration. Even though most 16:8 followers drink water during their fasting times, it may not be enough (food itself provides a little water).

There is a possibility of disordered eating habits as the result of intermittent fasting. According to studies, fasting for an amount of time followed by a small window of opportunity to eat primes you to overeat. It's a tough cycle to break because it interferes with the bodies' metabolism and natural hunger cues. Restricted eating can also improve the odds of developing anxiety and depression.

It is particularly concerning for women, who have a higher risk of developing eating disorders in the past. Binge-purge tendencies will (and should) occur due to allotted periods of restriction accompanied by feeding. According to the National Eating Disorders Association, binging and fasting periods are risk factors for eating disorders.

Should you try fasting for 16 hours?

In the end, it's a personal decision. However, then you can adopt healthy habits by sticking to the riskier aspects of 16-hour fasting. The first step is to learn more about mindfulness and how it applies to your eating habits. To get started, think about the following questions when determining when and what to eat:

Most of us eat based on circumstances rather than hunger levels. There are times you've ever gone to the cinema after dinner and found yourself craving popcorn?

You could notice patterns you didn't even notice before if you consider the times when you eat. Assume you enjoy grazing while watching The Bachelor. If you fast after 8 p.m., you've immediately cut hours off your post-dinner snacking — and therefore, calories.

If you stop late-night snacking, you might be able to go to bed sooner, which is a vital aspect of any weight-loss strategy. Sleeping for seven hours a night has been related to better weight control, a lower risk of chronic illness, and a faster metabolism.

3.3 5:2 fasting

It is a common intermittent fasting process that involves eating less than two days a week. This eating plan encourages you to eat regularly for five days and then seriously limit calories on 2 days of your choice.

Diets like the 5:2 diet appeal to many people who want to lose weight or boost their health because no foods are forbidden. However, since the 5:2 is one of the most restrictive types of intermittent fasting, some people may find it difficult to follow.

Expert Opinion: "The 5:2 diet is one of the most common intermittent diets, and you'll probably lose weight if you adopt it since you'll be eating fewer calories overall. It's a strict diet that can be difficult to stick to, particularly on intermittent fasting days" (Kelly Plowe, MS, RD).

THE 5:2 DIET

DAY 1	DAY 2	DAY 3	DAY 4	DAY 5	DAY 6	DAY 7
Eat normally	Women: 500 calories Men: 600 calories	Eat normally	Eat normally	Women: 500 calories Men: 600 calories	Eat normally	Eat normally

Background

Intermittent fasting has been practiced as a religious, spiritual, and political action for hundreds of years. Pythagoras, the Greek philosopher, fasted and urged others to do the same, as did the Renaissance and Hippocrates doctor Paracelsus.

Major religions around the world also observe sacred times. Muslims fast in the Holy month of Ramadan. Christians fast on several days during Lent, while those who practice Judaism observe many fasts during the year. Fasting has been used by political figures such as Mahatma Gandhi as a form of political protest.

Fasting has recently gained popularity as a means of improving one's health and fitness. Intermittent fasting has become the next big thing, following the keto, paleo, low-carb, and commercial diet patterns. Intermittent fasting can be done in various forms, including water fasting, warrior diet, and more.

Dr. Michael Mosley, a UK-based writer, wrote a book called The Easy Diet that popularized the 5:2 diet. Mosley received his medical training in London. In the novel, he sets out a strategy in which you fast for 2 days a week and eat normally eat rest of the time.

Benefits

With Intermittent fasting, there have been a few primary areas of scientific interest. Researchers have been looking at whether diets like the 5:2 diet can help people lose weight, control or avoid diabetes, and improve their heart health. The results of studies have been mixed, and study authors often state that conducting research is difficult.

"Medical evidence for the health benefits of intermittent fasting in humans is often extrapolated from animal studies, based on observational data on religious fasting (especially Ramadan), or derived from experimental studies with modest sample sizes", according to one researcher.

However, as the popularity of these programs has grown, further research has been performed.

The 5:2 diet, according to a new study published in The American Journal of Clinical Nutrition, is a viable choice for obese people trying to lose weight and improve their cardiovascular health. However, the study was limited in reach (16 participants) and lasted just 10 weeks.

Another research looked at the impact of intermittent fasting on diabetic study participants. The 5:2 diet was compared to daily calorie restriction in a long-term study published in JAMA.

For a year, five researchers followed 100 participants. One-third of the participants practiced the 5:2 diet, one-third followed a daily calorie reduction plan (75 percent of daily energy needs), and one-third did not make any dietary changes.

Of the three diet types, the 5:2 diet had the largest drop-out rate. Although both the daily calorie restriction and the 5:2 groups lost weight, the amount lost was not significantly different. Additionally, at six months and one year, there were no significant differences in fasting glucose, blood pressure, C-reactive protein, insulin resistance, fasting insulin, or homocysteine concentrations between the intervention groups. The 5:2 fasting group also had significantly higher levels of low-density lipoprotein cholesterol at the end of the analysis.

How Does It Work?

The 5:2 diet's simplicity is part of its appeal. You won't have to stick to any complex meal plans, and you won't have to weigh portions or count calories.

Duration

During the majority of the week, the 5:2 diet helps you to eat "normally." On 2 days of the week, you limit your calorie consumption.

On fasting days, the calorie consumption is limited to 500 calories for women and 600 calories for men (for men). You normally eat for the remaining five days. However, Mosley states in the book that eating "normally" means eating the number of calories the body requires to perform everyday functions (also known as total daily energy expenditure). That means you won't be able to eat too much on your non fasting days. Instead, you're advised to eat a variety of foods in reasonable portions.

What to Eat?

On the 5:2 diet, you are usually free to eat whatever you want. One of the key advantages of intermittent fasting is that there are no "good" or "bad" foods.

Instead of concentrating on food composition (such as how much calories or protein food contains), the 5:2 diet emphasizes meal timing.

On the other hand, on any eating plan, you can try to consume healthy foods. Vegetables, lean proteins, fruits, healthy fats and whole grains are the safest things to consume on the 5:2 diet. On fasting days, healthy fats and protein are particularly important because they provide your brain and body with extra energy.

To fill up space in the stomach on fasting days, continue to consume high-volume, low-calorie foods. Broccoli and carrots, which are high in fiber, are good options for keeping you full.

You can drink whatever you want on normal eating days, but you should adhere to water to stay under the calorie limit for that day on fasting days.

Compliant Foods

- Whole grains
- Vegetables
- Fruits
- High-fiber foods
- Healthy fats
- Lean protein

- Red meat
- Beverages

Whole grains: They are high in vitamins and fiber, keeping you feeling satisfied and full. Since quinoa, brown rice, pasta, whole-wheat bread, and other tasty grains are good for the brain, they are all included in the 5:2 diet.

Vegetables: Broccoli, leafy greens, cauliflower, sweet potatoes, Brussels sprouts, squash—the 5:2 diet allows for all of these vegetables and more. Fill the plate with a variety of colors to get a variety of good nutrients.

Fruits: Fruit is a nutritious addition to almost every diet. On the 5:2 diet, you will eat berries, starchy fruits, citrus fruits, and more.

High-fiber foods: Beans, lentils, legumes, oatmeal and sprouted grains are all high-fiber foods that will keep you full while also providing vital nutrients to your body, particularly on fasting days.

Healthy fats: Nuts, olive oil, seeds, fatty fish, avocados, and other forms of omega-3s and omega-6s can all be included in your 5:2 diet schedule. When your body's glycogen reserves run out, these will provide energy.

Lean protein: Chicken breast, chickens, ground turkey, and fish are high in lean protein, which your body needs for muscle growth and cellular repair. For better fitness, consider these lean protein choices.

Red meat: While it's best to eat more lean protein, a few servings of red meat per week won't hurt. Consider using lean ground beef or a lean steak cut.

Beverages: On normal days, you can drink anything you want, but on fasting days, it's best to stick to zero-calorie drinks. On low-calorie days, stick to black coffee, water, and herbal tea.

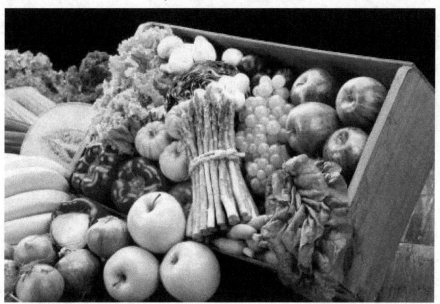

Non-compliant Foods
- Beverages other than water (on fasting days)
- No foods are technically off-limits

Recommended Timing

For the other 5 days of the week, eat normally. It doesn't mean you can eat more than usual to make up for the calories you've missed on fasting days. If you eat more on "regular" days to make up for the calories you've lost on fasting days, you may not lose weight. You can also gain weight if you consume too many high-calorie, high-sugar, or excessively refined foods regularly.

So do your best to make your days as normal as possible.

You should play with timing on fasting days to see what works best for your brain and body. Some people work better with a light breakfast, while others tend to delay their first meal as long as possible. You should strive to eat around 25% of the daily caloric intake.

Since you only have so many calories to deal with, you can spread them out as much as possible. Eating a lot of high-volume foods can help. If you want to eat 500 calories on the fasting day, you could eat 200 calories for breakfast, 100 calories for lunch, and then another 200 calories for dinner. Alternatively, you could eat 250 calories at lunch & 250 calories at dinner.

It is completely up to you to determine which fasting days you can follow. The schedule below is an example of a standard protocol:

- Sunday: normal
- Monday: fast
- Tuesday: normal
- Wednesday: normal
- Thursday: fast
- Friday: normal
- Saturday: normal

Resources and Tips

If you've never fasted before, there's a fair chance you'll experience side effects on fasting days. Fasting has the following side effects:

- Fatigue
- Hunger
- Mood swings
- Irritability
- Nausea
- Headaches
- Weakness
- Trouble focusing
- Loss of productivity
- Sleepiness

These are common side effects of fasting, and they normally go away once the body gets used to it. If you're feeling hungry, irritability, or some of the other side effects, consider the following methods to help them pass:

- Stay busy with work or errands
- Drink more water
- Meditate
- Take a nap
- Take a shower or bath
- Take a stretch break
- Call a friend

The bulk of the fasting side effects will fade away if you stop worrying about them. Fasting can become second nature to your body over time.

Modifications

It's not easy to go from eating normally every day to just eating 500–600 calories twice a week. Instead of making such a drastic change, gradually reduce the calorie intake on fasting days. Reduce the consumption from 2000 to up to 1500 calories over the first week, for example. Try eating just 1000 calories the next week. After that, reduce the calories in small amounts until you're consuming the 500–600 calories recommended on fasting days.

Chapter No 4: Practical tips for Intermittent Fasting

4.1 Intermittent Fasting - Tips for Success

Have you heard about the new diet craze, intermittent fasting? There's a reason why so many actors do it, and so many people have succeeded in it. This diet isn't a diet at all; when practiced correctly, it can become a habit. Don't be deceived by out-of-date diets like skipping meals; we all know they don't work. Intermittent fasting does not suggest missing meals, counting calories, or seriously restricting the diet (what a relief!). It means that you want to eat within a certain time frame while fasting for the rest of the time. It's important to remember that this isn't about starvation but rather about splitting the calories differently.

Intermittent fasting will help you lose weight while also lowering your blood pressure, improving glucose levels, and even slowing down the aging process (yes, this is a thing). When we eat, our insulin levels rise, converting to stored sugar in the liver and causes fat to develop. When we fast, our insulin levels drop and burn off the sugar that's accumulated. To put it another way, if you are always eating, your body will use the food as energy, which means you will never burn the fat you have stored in the body.

Diets can be difficult to follow, take time away from your life, restrict you, and be very expensive. Fasting, on the other hand, lets you simplify your life and is healthy. It saves you time by enabling you to cook fewer meals, and it is available to you at any time and from any place. There are several strong reasons to begin this diet and make it a habit. Of course, before making any big lifestyle changes, you should consult a doctor! When you're ready to give intermittent fasting a try, here are ten tips to get you started!

1. Pick the Fasting Time for You

Since the intermittent quick is so adaptable, you must select a style that will work for you. It can be followed in a variety of ways. You have the choice of using the 16:8 or 20:4 method. The 16:8 approach entails fasting for 16 hours a day (a large portion of which will be spent sleeping), followed by an 8-hour window for eating. A 4-hour eating window follows a 20-hour fast in the 20:4 method. Both of these plans give you the freedom to begin and end them whenever you like. You might break your fast at noon and eat until 8 p.m. If breakfast is more significant to you and you have the strength to avoid evening snacking, a 10 a.m. to 6 p.m. window could be more suitable.

You may also opt for a longer fasting time. It can include the 5:2 diet, which involves eating five days a week and fasting for two days. This diet is so adaptable that you can pick whatever works for you or is more practical while still getting the same results.

2. Start Gradually

When beginning a new lifestyle or diet, such as intermittent fasting, slow and steady pace is recommended. It will assist the body in adapting to a more smooth transition. If fasting from your usual breakfast time until noon does not work for you, consider increasing it by one hour the first day and two hours the day after until you can go until lunchtime without eating.

Some people will jump straight into something different and push through the difficult times and cravings, but if you're not one of them, you should start gradually if you want to see results.

3. Survive the Hunger Waves

Hunger isn't constant; it comes in waves. The next time you feel like you can't take it any longer, consider riding out the hunger wave. Contrary to common opinion, once you get hungry, it won't keep building up until you feel like you're going to explode; it will finally subside, and all you have to do now is get through it.

When hunger strikes, it's important to stay hydrated. Your body may be displaying signs of hunger as a result of dehydration when all you need is some water!

4. Drink a lot of water

As previously mentioned, it is important to drink a lot of water while fasting. It not only keeps you hydrated but also makes your stomach feel full. You are free to drink as much water as you want. Drinking coffee or tea (but only black; sugar and cream will break your fast) will also help fulfill any cravings you might have during your fasting period.

5. Don't Binge

When fasting, this is extremely important. Make every attempt to stop breaking your fast by overeating. When breaking your fast, it can be difficult not to reach for the largest meal you can find, especially in the beginning. If you do, you risk eating too quickly, too much, and making poor food decisions, all of which will make your body hate you later. When it comes to breaking your fast, the safest thing to do is schedule out healthier foods to eat and eat slowly. Begin with a light meal, and if you get hungry again quickly, try a different snack.

6. Eat Wholesome Meals

It may seem obvious, but make sure you're filling your body with healthy foods in between fasting times. According to some research, eating a low-carb diet during intermittent fasting will make you feel less hungry. Not to mention that consuming nutritious foods helps the body feel healthy and gives your mind the energy it needs to think clearly. We've all had the experience of eating a fast food meal that leaves you with a sense of brain fog and makes your body feel demotivated and heavy for the rest of the day.

7. Stay Busy

Keeping active is one of the most effective ways to relieve yourself from what might seem to be hunger. How much of you notice yourself eating unnecessarily when bored? It is when you have plenty to consume your mind, so you say, "Oh, I'm starving," though you aren't. To keep yourself busy, try taking up a new hobby. Reading a book, listening to a podcast, or even cleaning the house will all help. Perhaps better, get that butt moving and do a workout to hold yourself occupied. Nothing beats adding at least 30 minutes of exercise into your day to promote a healthier lifestyle, not to mention the fact that it can keep you away from calories and helping you feel amazing. If you can't stop worrying about food at work, rethink your task. Perhaps you should take a 5-minute break to change tasks; the important thing is to keep occupied, so that thoughts about food don't stick in your head and take you off track.

8. Journal

It is a wonderful and essential tip, journal! From the start, keep track of everything. If you're a tech person, use your phone, but keep a record in a journal if you're more traditional.

Keeping track of your everyday food consumption during non-fasting hours is a smart thing, as is keeping track of your moods, both good and bad, in the process. This way, you'll be able to see how far you've progressed. It could have been your body getting accustomed to the fresh fasting you've been trying, or it could have been the big bun you had for lunch that made you furious on Monday afternoon. If you don't track your weight loss or healthier lifestyle journey, it's difficult to know any patterns. Take a lot of photographs in addition to tracking moods and food consumption. Seeing is the simplest way to believe. Take before and after pictures because you have plenty to look back on and see if you've achieved some progress.

9. Get Rid of the Negative People

It's vital to say the right people whether you're following a fresh diet or something you're particularly enthusiastic about. Whether you have many bad people in your life or knowing someone has negative feelings, don't carry them out on your new adventure. When beginning a new diet or lifestyle, it is important to have the correct support net. To help you succeed, you'll need others to assist you, inspire you, and support your new path.

10. Wait For at least a month

The most important thing to note before initiating every new routine or activity is to allow it time. The proverb "Rome wasn't built in a day" has a lot of significance. You can't hope to lose a lot of weight by doing intermittent fasting for a few days. It takes time for your body to adapt, and it takes time for your mind to make it a habit. If you're planning to pursue intermittent fasting, give it at least a month before deciding if it's right for you.

4.2 Awareness

It works best if you stop feeding at a specific time of day and don't eat at all at night. That implies no snacks in between or before bed. While feeding times vary from person to person, people improve eating between 10 a.m. and 6 p.m.

Is it tough to follow?

Intermittent fasting may be challenging at first; however, when the body adjusts to a different way of eating, the diet becomes more manageable. The end goal is to become more conscious about what and when you consume. It establishes limits and boundaries, which many of my patients appreciate. The regular workout is promoted, avoiding sugars, and consuming vegetables, fruits, lentils, beans, lean proteins, whole grains, and healthy fats in addition to intermittent fasting.

When is the most effective time to fast?

Fat burning usually starts after 12 hours of fasting and increases between 16 and 24 hours of fasting.

How many days a week is this fasting recommended?

People usually fast for up to 16 hours a day. It is normally accomplished by missing breakfast the next morning after consuming the previous day's final meal. Intermittent fasting is a pattern that entails going without eating for 24 hours up to two days per week.

What is the maximum amount of food that can be consumed during the eating period?

If you choose to lose weight, stick to a calorie intake that allows you to lose one to two pounds every week. You'll need to eat off 500 calories a day on average to drop one pound per week.

Is there some beverage that you should drink during the fast?

Water, and plenty of it. If you're going to fast, make sure you drink plenty of water during the period you're not consuming solid food. Broth made from vegetables, chicken, or bone broth may also be eaten. Caffeine-containing beverages and soda can be avoided.

Are there any other benefits of intermittent fasting besides weight loss?

Fasting can help improve glucose control, lower cholesterol, improve blood pressure, reduce liver fat, and reducing body weight. Patients report greater endurance, improved motor coordination, and better sleep. Eating under the circadian cycle (eat during the day, sleep at night) helps promote deep sleep. Fasting, which results in caloric restriction, has also been found to prolong the lifespan of even healthier people in research. According to studies, fasting has also been related to a decrease in tumor growth and the prevention of breast cancer recurrence.

Does it involve calorie counting?

Not actually, but if you skip snacks before bedtime and go longer hours without feeding, the calorie intake can decrease. You're still eating things that are usually lower in calories while you eat a mostly plant-based diet.

Who is the most benefited from intermittent fasting?

Intermittent fasting isn't suitable for anyone. It is another item to include in the toolkit for those who have tried to lose weight. In the end, it comes down to a person's lifestyle and the decisions he or she makes. They must assess their choices and determine what would be better for them?

Is there any reason to avoid intermittent fasting if you have a medical condition?

People with brittle diabetes, people with a history of eating problems such as bulimia and anorexia, and breastfeeding or pregnant women do not fast unless a doctor closely monitors them.

4.3 Understanding the Body Mass Index

If your BMI is less than 18.5 points, you are considered underweight. Please remember that a BMI calculation that is too low will result in health problems. For more details on BMI estimates, please contact your healthcare provider.

If your BMI is about 18.5-24.9, you have a regular BMI. This healthier weight lowers the chances of major health problems and indicates that you're close to achieving your wellness goals.

If your BMI is between 25 and 29.9, you are considered overweight. Overweight people are more likely to experience cardiovascular disease. To boost your health, consult the healthcare professional and start implementing lifestyle improvements such as healthier eating and exercise.

If your BMI is greater than 30, you are considered obese. Obese people are more likely to experience various diseases and health issues, including cardiovascular disease, high blood pressure (hypertension), Type 2 diabetes, breathing problems, and more. To boost your physical health and quality of life, visit the healthcare provider and start implementing lifestyle improvements such as healthier eating and exercise.

4.4 Possible Downsides of IF, if not followed properly

Some programs may cause more side effects than others, so it's important to speak to a doctor about the following intermittent fasting side effects before deciding on a plan that suits your lifestyle.

1. Intermittent fasting can make you sick.

People may experience lethargy, headaches, constipation, and crankiness depending on how long they fast. You may want to shift from alternate day fasting to a time-restricted feeding plan or periodic fasting that requires you to eat every day within a certain period to minimize any of these unwanted side effects.

2. It can lead to overeating.

Since your appetite hormones and hunger center in your brain go into full force when deprived of food, there is a strong biological push to overeat after fasting times.

"Its human nature to want to reward themselves after performing very hard work, like exercise or fasting for a lengthy amount of time, so there's a risk of indulging in unhealthy eating patterns on non-fasting days," — Dr. Frank Hu, chair of the Harvard T.H. Chan School of Public Health's nutrition department.

According to a report in 2018, 2 common side effects of calorie-restricted diets—increased appetite and slowed metabolism —can occur when people practice intermittent fasting when they reduce calorie intake every day. And the evidence is clear in studies of time-restricted feeding that eating that is out of alignment with a person's circadian rhythm (their body's normal daily pattern) can lead to metabolic issues.

3. Intermittent fasting in older adults may result in excessive weight loss.

Although intermittent fasting has shown promise, there is still less evidence about its benefits or how it can affect older people. Small groups of young or middle-aged adults have been studied in humans for only brief periods.

However, we do know that intermittent fasting can be harmful in some situations. Losing too much weight can affect your overall immune system, bones, and energy level.

4. It may be dangerous if you're taking certain medications.

Dr. Eric Rimm advises that you first talk to a doctor if you want to try intermittent fasting. For people with certain diseases, such as diabetes, severely limiting calories and skipping meals may be harmful. Some people who take blood pressure or heart disease medications may be more prone to potassium, sodium, and other mineral imbalances during longer-than-normal fasting periods.

"People who need to take their drugs with food — to prevent stomach irritation or nausea — do not do well with fasting," says Dr. Suzanne Salamon.

4.5 Reducing the Harmful Effects of Intermittent Fasting

Easing into a fasting schedule will help the body adapt. For several months, gradually reduce the time window for feeding. It would help if you also kept taking your medications as prescribed by your doctor. Drink calorie-free drinks like water or black coffee to stay hydrated. If you need to take medicine with food, use a revised fasting plan approved by the doctor.

When you're fasting, keep yourself busy. When you're new to IF, it's weird not to eat! You might discover that eating (especially snacking) is now a habit, so keep yourself occupied during your fasting window to ensure you don't surrender to temptation. If you're not at work, find a hobby, spend time with friends, or read a book to keep yourself busy.

4.6 Meal Plan for Intermediate Fasting

This plan allows you to eat only between 12 p.m. and 6 p.m. for a total of 18 hours of fasting over 24 hours.

If you don't eat breakfast, it's still important to keep hydrated. Make sure you continue to drink plenty of water. Herbal tea is also a choice (most experts agree that coffee and tea do not break a fast.) Tea catechism have been shown to increase the benefits of fasting by lowering the hunger hormone ghrelin, allowing you to go until lunch without feeling deprived.

Since you've added four hours to your fasting time, make sure the first meal (at noon) contains enough healthy fats. The burger from the 8-to-6-window plan will work great, and you can improve the fat content with the dressing or avocado on top!

Seeds and nuts are rich-fat snacks that can be consumed at 2:30 p.m. Soaking them ahead of time will help neutralize enzymes that occur naturally, like phytates, which can cause digestive problems. Dinner should be at 5:30 p.m., and, as with the 8 -6 window schedule, a dinner of healthy protein source with vegetables or wild-caught fish is a great choice.

- First meal: Grass-fed burger with avocado at noon.
- Snack: Seeds and Nuts at 2:30 p.m.
- Second meal: Veggies and Salmon at 5:30 p.m.

The 2-day meal plan

Eat clean for five days a week as part of this program (you can pick whatever days you want). Limit the calories to no more than 700 a day on the other two days. Calorie restriction offers many of the same advantages as a full-day fast.

On non-fasting days, make sure you're getting enough lean meats, healthy fats, fruits and vegetables, and you can structure your meals however suits you best.

On restricted days, you can eat smaller meals or snacks during the day or eat a moderate lunch and dinner while fasting throughout the morning and after dinner. Eat lean meats, healthy fats, and fresh produce. Apps will help you manage your meals and keep track of the calorie intake to exceed 700 calories.

The 5-2 meal plan (advanced).

You'll eat clean five days a week on this plan, but you won't eat anything for 2 nonconsecutive days. On Mondays and Thursdays, you can fast but eat clean meals on the other days. These five days' food will be similar to the rest of the fasting plans, consisting of healthy fats, lean meat sources, vegetables, and fruit.

This plan is not for beginners, and you should always consult your doctor before beginning any fasting regimen, particularly if you are taking medication or have a medical condition. Coffee drinkers should maintain their morning coffee consumption, and anyone doing an advanced quick should remain well hydrated.

- Monday is a fast day.
- Tuesday: Include healthy fats, lean meat, vegetables, and fruit in your diet.
- Wednesday: Include healthy fats, vegetables, lean meat, and fruit in your diet.
- Thursday is a fast day.
- Friday: Include healthy fats, vegetables, lean meat, and fruit in your diet.
- Saturday: Include healthy fats, vegetables, lean meat, and fruit in your diet.

5. Advanced: Alternate-day fasting or an every-other-day schedule.

Despite its advancement, this method is very easy to implement. Every other day, don't eat anything.

Eat clean meat sources, healthy fats, vegetables, and some fruit every other day, and then only water, herbal tea, and moderate quantities of black coffee or tea on fasting days.

- Monday: Include healthy fats, lean meat, vegetables, and berries in your diet.

- Tuesday is a fast day.

- Wednesday: Include healthy fats, vegetables, lean meat, and fruit in your diet.

- Thursday is a fast day.

- Friday: Include healthy fats, vegetables, lean meat, and berries in your diet.

- Saturday is a fast day.

- Sunday: Include healthy fats, vegetables, lean meat, and fruit in your diet.

With this experience, you should be able to schedule your meals precisely when beginning an intermittent fasting program. And, while it may appear difficult at first, once you get into the habit of fasting, it will feel natural and fit into your daily routine. However, you should always begin slowly and work your way up to more advanced plans.

It's also important to keep in mind that intermittent fasting will not work for you on certain days. Listen to your body—fine, it's if you need to eat outside of your usual window. Restart when you're in a better mood.

4.7 Working Out and Intermittent Fasting

Working out before breakfast is another way of implying you exercise while on an intermittent fast. An intermittent fast is when your body goes without food for a while (including while you're sleeping) over 24 hours. The IF window starts when you take your last bite of food or drink (apart from water) before going to bed and finishes when you take the first bite of food the next day.

The duration of the intermittent fast must be between 16 and 18 hours to reap the most benefits. Eat-in between the hours of 10:30 a.m. & 6:30 p.m.

When Do You Work out When Intermittent Fasting?

The optimal time to exercise during intermittent fasting is usually right after waking up or shortly after. It helps to support the body's normal circadian rhythm. Working out (or eating) too close to bedtime has been shown to disrupt deep and REM sleep levels, so save the workout for the next day.

You shouldn't eat right after a workout for the same reasons you shouldn't eat right after a fasted workout: hormone optimization. According to research, waiting two to three hours after a workout before eating encourages increased growth hormone, which aids in fat burning and energy replacement (sugar). A hormone change occurs as a result of adaptation to the stress induced by a high-intensity exercise. If your schedule only allows for a lunchtime workout, you can exercise during that time and then enjoy the hormonal benefits of not eating for two to three hours afterward.

Intermittent Fasting and Cardio

The hormonal benefits of fasting-induced exercise are linked to the depletion of muscle and liver glycogen stores when you fast. It's good to do cardio when intermittent fasting, but the results will be dictated by how fat-adapted your body is (how good it is at burning fat for fuel instead of glucose). You should expect a slight decrease in results if you're new to fasting and exercise; it can take up to six months for some athletes to completely adapt their fitness to this new fuel source. If you're a professional athlete, for example, and your primary objective is to boost your race results, don't turn to fasted training a few weeks before a competition. If you're doing cardio when fasting, don't keep the fast running after the workout; instead, refill afterward.

Intermittent Fasting and Sprint Training

High-intensity interval training (aka HIIT) or Sprint training involves intervals of intense activity accompanied by rest for around 15 to 30 minutes. Not only is sprint training time effective, but studies show that it has health benefits that aerobic exercise alone cannot provide, such as a substantial increase in human growth hormone (HGH). Sprint training has many advantages, including enhanced muscle and brain strength and endurance, increased growth hormone, improved body structure, improved brain function, higher testosterone levels, and reduced depression. Many of these advantages are improved when sprint training is combined with intermittent fasting. Sprint training is an excellent way to integrate exercise into your fasting time, and you can stretch your fast two to three hours afterward to gain even more benefits.

Weightlifting and Fasting

Weightlifting while fasting is also normal, but you should be aware of the role sugar plays in muscle repair after a big weightlifting exercise, particularly while fasting. Your glycogen reserves are already exhausted when you perform exercise during fasting. If your day's workout includes heavy lifting, it can be done while fasting; however, you should eat a meal right afterward. Unlike a quick workout session, heavy lifting imposes enough stress on the body to require an immediate refeed. Lifting weights while fasting, like cardio, can reduce the strength in the short term as the body adjusts to being a "fat burner." As a result, you may want to reserve the weightlifting sessions for once you've eaten (in which scenario you can fast for 2 to 3 hours afterward) and include fasted exercise on days when you do burst-style training.

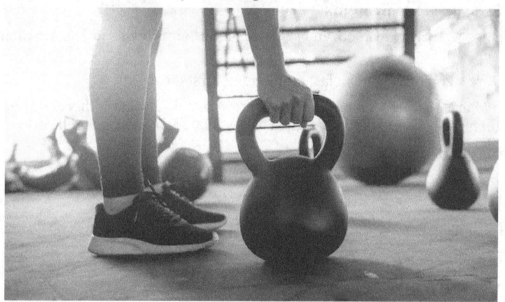

Fasting while exercising is appropriate and helpful for hormone optimization (which is the secret to a variety of health benefits, including better body composition). Combining burst training and intermittent fasting for a multi-therapeutic strategy will maximize the advantages of both.

Weight training and cardio can also be done in a fasting state, but the performance may suffer a little. Early in the day is the best time to exercise when fasting to adjust the body's natural circadian rhythm; but, whether you're doing endurance cardio or a heavyweight session, you can still gain hormonal benefits from fasting after the workout (for 2 to 3 hours).

CHAPTER No 5: Shopping list to prepare for Intermittent Fasting

5.1 Best Food to Break an Intermittent Fast

On the intermittent fasting diet, you can eat the following three foods:

Although Bulletproof Coffee is a good way to break the fast, you should also consider consuming other foods to help you break the Intermittent Fasting period.

To get the most out of IF, make sure you get the majority of your calories from nutrient-dense foods throughout your "feeding" windows. Learn about fasting & feeding windows in this chapter.

Choose whole foods to make healthy meals that can keep you energized and help the body absorb nutrients more efficiently during fasts.

Using healthy fats to break the fast

Bulletproof coffee, grass-fed butter, coffee, seeds, nuts, butter, nuts, coconut oil, olive oil, and avocados are excellent healthy-fat choices for breaking your fast.

Eat Complex Carbohydrates

Sweet potatoes, rice, white potatoes, oats, quinoa, and other whole grains are all important.

To break your fast, you should avoid high-sugar foods instead of concentrating on healthy fats and proteins. To put it another way, skip the cereal and go for scrambled eggs or an omelet instead.

Break the fast with lean proteins

Chicken, beef, pork, turkey, seafood, and eggs are important proteins to include when breaking a fast.

Mini quiches are a great choice for a fast grab-and-go first meal.

According to Maciel, eating lean protein allows you to feel full than other foods and helps you sustain or gain muscle. Here are five protein sources that are both lean and healthy:

- Plain Greek yogurt.
- Chicken breast.
- Tofu and tempeh.
- Fish and shellfish.
- Beans, peas and lentils.

Eat one serving of fruit

A serving of fruit, whether fresh or frozen, is a tasty way to get micronutrients. To keep the blood sugar levels stable, limit yourself to one serving.

Due to the concentrated amount of sugars per serving, canned fruits and juice should be avoided.

Fruits

Intermittent fasting, like every other eating plan, requires the consumption of high-nutrient foods. Vitamins, minerals, phytonutrients (plant nutrients), and fiber are commonly found in fruits and vegetables. These vitamins, minerals, and nutrients can reduce cholesterol, blood sugar regulation, and bowel health. Another advantage is the low-calorie level in fruits and vegetables.

According to the government's Dietary Guidelines for Americans, most people should consume about 2 cups of fruit a day on a 2,000-calorie diet.

Here are ten good fruits to eat while fasting intermittently:

- Watermelon.
- Apricots.
- Oranges.
- Blueberries.
- Plums.
- Blackberries.
- Pears.
- Apples.
- Cherries.
- Peaches.

Eat all the veggies you want

I'm sure you already know this, but breaking the fast with a large serving of vegetables is always a good idea.

If you don't have time to prepare a meal, a Green Pineapple Smoothie to-go or a Blueberry Muffin Smoothie are great options. Both have a good amount of greens and are nutrient-dense.

Vegetables

Vegetables will help you stick to your intermittent fasting plan. A diet high in leafy greens has been shown to lower the risk of Type 2 diabetes, heart disease, cognitive decline, cancer, and other diseases. According to the government's Dietary Guidelines for Americans, most people should consume 2.5 cups of vegetables a day on a 2,000-calorie diet.

Here are 6 vegetables that would be beneficial to include in a balanced intermittent eating plan:

- Cabbage.
- Kale.
- Arugula.
- Spinach.
- Chard.
- Collard greens.

5.2 Foods to Avoid

Certain foods should not be consumed as part of the intermittent fasting regimen. Avoid foods that are high in sugar, fat, and salt and are high in calories. "They won't satisfy you after a short, and they might even make you hungry," Maciel says. "They also don't provide much in the form of nutrients."

Avoid the following foods if you want to stick to an intermittent eating plan:

- Microwave popcorn.
- Snack chips.

Foods with a lot of added sugar can also be avoided. According to Maciel, sugar in processed foods and beverages is devoid of nutrients and amounts to empty calories, sweet, which you don't want if you're intermittently fasting. "Because sugar metabolizes so quickly, they'll make you hungry," he says.

If you're doing intermittent fasting, stay away from sugary foods like:

- Cookies.

- Sugary cereals and granola.

- Candy.

- Fruit juice.

- Cakes.

- Barbecue sauce and ketchup.

5.3 The Best Foods to Eat When You're Intermittently Fasting

Intermittent fasting has risen to the top of the list of diets for women over 50. It also doesn't need costly cookbooks, time-consuming manuals, or even a specialized trainer or dietician, in addition to its anti-aging and weight-loss results. However, it's also important to note that the foods you consume while intermittent fasting are just as important as the timing of the fast. Continue reading to discover the best foods to consume for intermittent fasting to maintain better health and weight loss. First and foremost—make a schedule for your intermittent fasting.

The 16:8 Intermittent Fasting schedule works better for women. However, since everybody is different, you might find that a different schedule is more suitable. Before reading more about the healthiest meals for intermittent fasting, take a look at these other fasting schedules:

- Alternate Day Fasting (ADF) consists of ad libitum eating one day, followed by one day of full fasting.

- Modified Alternate Day Fasting (mADF) involves one day of usual eating with a low-calorie diet one day (about 25% of regular caloric intake).

- 2/5: Two days of complete fasting followed by 5 days of ad libitum feeding;

- 1/6: Full fasting for 1 day of the week, then eating normally the rest of the week;

- Fasting for 12-20 hours a day (as a continuation of the nighttime fast) on every day of the week with an "eating window" of 4-12 hours is known as Time Restricting Feeding (TRF).

Below are the best foods to consume during intermittent fasting:

Water

If you're going without food for an extended period, hydration becomes even more important. When you fast, the sugar stored in the liver becomes the body's preferred energy source (glycogen). You lose a large number of electrolytes and fluid as you burn this energy. As a result, it's important to consume at least 8 cups of water a day. Not only can this avoid dehydration, but it will also improve blood flow, joint and muscle support, and cognitive function.

Grains that are minimally processed

Carbs, whether you like them or not, are a necessary part of life. It's also important to consider how to strategically consume enough calories without being too full and satisfied while fasting.

Choose foods that are easy to digest, such as crackers and whole-grain bread. These will also provide an excellent source of energy when on the go.

Coffee

If you've been putting off starting this diet because you can't live without coffee, there's good news. Coffee is a calorie-free drink in its natural state, so you can drink it even if you're fasting! Leave out the creamers, syrups, and other flavors.

Lentils

Half a cup of lentils provides about a third of the regular fiber requirements! They're also high in iron (approximately 15% of your daily requirement), so women can eat plenty of them!

Raspberries

Looking for a tasty way to increase your fiber intake? Go for the raspberries. These berries have eight grams of fiber per cup, which lets you consume more whole fruits.

Hummus

For those who are intermittently fasting, this creamy, delicious dip is a perfect plant-based protein. It also works well as a mayonnaise replacement. Hummus is a perfect mini-meal to consume during the middle of your 8-hour eating window in the 16:8 intermittent fast.

Potatoes

White potatoes, like our minimally processed grains, are relatively easy to digest. You should combine them with a source of protein for a post-workout meal to refuel your muscles if you're exercising and intermittent fasting. Another advantage of including potatoes in your IF diet is that they create a resistant starch that fuels your gut bacteria when they cool.

Salmon from the wild

With a shorter meal window, it's more important than ever to make sure you're getting enough vitamins and minerals from every bite! It's rich in the omega-3 fatty acids EPA and DHA, which are good for the brain. Serve it with your favorite roasted vegetables for a simple (and delicious) super food dinner.

Milk with added vitamin D

Adults require approximately 1,000 milligrams of calcium per day, which is about 3 glasses of milk. Although most people do not drink 3 glasses of milk a day, high-calcium foods should also be prioritized. It's great to add in smoothies or cereal. If you're lactose intolerant, go for tofu & leafy greens, just like kale.

Nuts

Nut intake was linked to a lower risk of Type 2 diabetes, cardiovascular disease, and overall mortality in a prospective trial published in the British Journal of Nutrition. So keep some in your pocket and use them when you're in the middle of your feeding window.

Chapter No 6: Tips and Tricks to Get Started on Intermittent Fasting

6.1 Remember To Drink Plenty of Water

When many people think of dieting, they generally think of losing weight. They do not eat or drink anything when they are thinking about losing the weight. It is unhealthy in any of the diet, but especially when intermittent fasting. That's because intermittent fasting isn't short-termed diet fad. It's something of a long-term shift in eating habits. Therefore, As a result, it's important to ensure that you're getting enough water daily during intermittent fasting. "Keeping the intake of water high helps in keeping the body's cells working and also the appetite under control," says Maya F. Bach. As a result, it's important to drink regularly during the day.

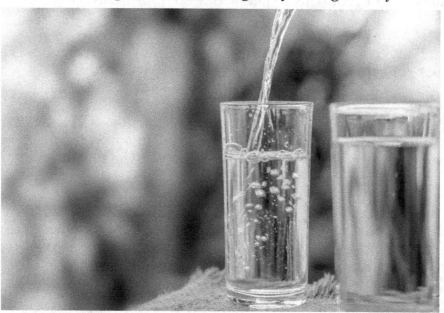

How much water is enough?

Drink half the weight of the body in ounces of water, according to a simple formula. If you weigh 180 pounds, then you can drink a minimum 90 ounces of water per day.

6.2 Avoid Eating Unhealthy Foods

One of most common mistakes people make when intermittent fasting focuses purely on eating rather than what to eat.

Just because you eat for eight hours a day doesn't mean you can eat whatever you want. "Those experimenting with intermittent fasting still need the same basic nutrients," says Whitney Linsenmyer, spokeswoman for the Academy of Nutrition and Dietetics. It's important to concentrate on consuming nutritious, healthy foods during intermittent fasting.

So If you usually eat junk food a lot and still want to intermittent fast, you'll have to avoid eating unhealthy foods. However, stopping right away can be difficult for you.

Instead of making a full 180-degree lifestyle change all at once, concentrate on slowly reducing fast food and gradually adding healthy alternatives. You'll be less likely to quit if you do this. Artificially flavored drinks should be avoided. Although it is important to remain hydrated while intermittent fasting, this does not mean you should drink every single thing. In reality, even though they claim to be low in sugar, it is critical to avoid chemically flavored drinks like energy drinks & sodas. They are commonly filled with artificial sweeteners which are bad for health (thus defeating the point of starting a healthy diet from beginning!) and make you much hungrier! As a result, instead of sticking to the diet, you can find yourself incapable to control and begin overeating!

6.3 Reduce Sugar Consumption As Much As Possible

Start reducing the sugar consumption with these tips:

- Toss the brown and white sugar, honey, syrup, and molasses together. Reduce the amount of sugar added to drinks and foods you consume daily, such as pancakes, cereal, coffee, and tea. Reduce the quantity of sugar you use by half & gradually reduce from there.

- Replace the drink with something else. Water is best, but diet drinks are a better option than sugary drinks if you want something sweet to drink or lose weight.

- Fruits may be eaten fresh, dried, frozen, or canned. Choose fruit that has been canned in water or natural juice. Fruit canned in syrup, particularly heavy syrup, should be avoided. To remove any excess syrup or juice, rinse and drain in a colander.

- Examine food labels and select items with the fewest added sugars. Sugars (natural) can be found in dairy and fruit products. The product's ingredients list will show you whether there are any added sugars.

- Add any fruit. Please do not add sugar to oatmeal or cereal. Try fresh fruit (strawberries, cherries or bananas) or dried fruit (cranberries, apricots or raisins).

- Reduce the amount of sugar called for in the recipe by one-third to one-half when baking cookies, brownies, or cakes. Often, you won't be able to tell the difference.

- Take a look at extracts. Using extracts like orange, vanilla, almond, or lemon instead of sugar in recipes.

- It should be replaced. Spices, rather than sugar, can be used to improve foods. Spices such as cinnamon, allspice, ginger, and nutmeg can be used.

- Make a substitution. In recipes, replace sugar with unsweetened applesauce (use equivalent amounts) and avoid non-nutritive sweeteners. Non-nutritive sweeteners can be a temporary cure for satisfying the sweet tooth if you're trying to lose weight. But be careful! Make sure that substituting non-nutritive sweeteners for sugary choices does not result in you consuming more lately.

6.4 Avoid Stress

Allow yourself to ease into it. When it comes to intermittent fasting, most people make the mistake of going -in immediately. Many people feel that the shock and challenge of adjusting to this modern method of eating are too much for them, and they stick to the old habits. It isn't going to work. Intermittent fasting should not be considered as diet but somewhat as way of life. As a result, it is preferable to ease into something if it means it will be further successful than jumping all in and failing. E.g., if you've decided to follow the 16/8 method, instead of skipping breakfast entirely and waiting until lunch, postpone breakfast by thirty minutes on the first day. Every day, postpone breakfast a little longer until you're just feeding at lunchtime. Intermittent fasting can be made much easier with little tricks just like this. You are much more likely to thrive if you make intermittent fasting your routine rather than diet.

1. Exercise

Regular exercise is one of most effective ways to calm the body and mind. Plus, exercise will lift your mood. However, for it to pay off, you must do it often.

So, how much exercise should you do each week?

Work up to 2 hrs & 30 mins of moderately intense exercise, such as brisk walks, or 75 minutes of intensive exercise, such as swimming laps, jogging, or engaging in other sports.

Focus on setting realistic fitness goals, so you don't give up. Above all, note that any workout is better than not doing at all.

2. Relax Your Muscles

Your muscles tense up when you're nervous. You will help loosen them up and refresh the body on your own by doing the following:

- Enjoying a massage
- Stretching
- Getting a good night's sleep
- Taking a hot bath or shower

3. Deep Breathing

Taking a few deep breaths and stopping. It will immediately relieve stress. When you get the hang of it, you'll be shocked by how much better you feel. Simply obey these five steps:

- Sit with your hands on the lap and the feet on the floor in a relaxed position. You may also lay down.
- Close the eyes.
- Imagine yourself in a relaxing place. It could be on the beach, in a lovely field of grass, or somewhere else that makes you feel calm.
- Slowly inhale and exhale deeply. Do this for 5 to 10 minutes.

4. Eat Well

Eating a regular, well-balanced diet will help you feel better in general. It may also help control your moods. Your meals should be full of vegetables, fruit, whole grains, and lean protein for energy. And don't skip any. It's not good for you and can put you in a bad mood, which can increase your stress.

5. Slow Down

Modern life is so hectic that we need to take a break to relax and enjoy. Analyze your life for small chances to do so. Set your clock 5 to 10 minutes ahead. You'll be able to arrive a little sooner and escape the burden of being late. Switch to the slow lane if you're driving on the highway to avoid road rage.

Break down large projects into smaller chunks. If you don't have to, don't try to respond to all 100 emails; instead, respond to a few of them.

6. Take a Break

To give your mind a break from stress, schedule some real downtime. It could be challenging for you at first if you are someone who loves setting goals. But if you stick with it, you'll come to enjoy these moments. You should relax by doing the following:

- Prayer
- Yoga
- Meditation
- Spending time in nature
- Tai chi
- Listening to the favorite music

7. Make Time for Hobbies

You must plan time for events that you enjoy. Every day, try to do something that makes you happy, and it will help you relax. It doesn't have to take a long time; 15 to 20 minutes will work. Hobbies that are relaxing include:

- Playing golf
- Reading
- Doing puzzles
- Knitting
- Watching a movie
- Doing an art project
- Playing board games and cards

8. Talk about Your Problems

If something is disturbing you, talking about it will help you relax. Family members, friends, a trusted clergyman, the doctor, or a therapist are all excellent choices. You can also interact with yourself. It's known as self-talk, and we all indulge in it. However, for self-talk to be beneficial in reducing tension, it must be positive rather than negative. So, when you're nervous, pay attention to what you're thinking or doing. Change the negative message you're sending yourself to a positive one. Don't tell yourself, "I can't do this," for example. Instead, tell yourself, "I can do this," or "I'm doing the best I can."

9. Don't Be So Hard On Yourself

Accept that no matter how hard you try, you will never be able to achieve perfection. You still don't have full control of your life. So, do yourself a favor and avoid overestimating your abilities. Often, remember to maintain your sense of humor. Laughter is one of the most powerful ways to relax.

10. Eliminate the Triggers

Determine the primary sources of stress in your life. Is it your career, your commute, or your schoolwork that's the problem? If you can figure out what they are, consider if you can get rid of them or at least reduce them in your life. If you're having trouble figuring out what's causing your tension, consider keeping a stress journal. Make a note of when you feel the most anxious to see if you can detect a pattern, then figure out how to avoid or reduce those triggers.

6.5 The Science of Sleep and Fasting

A body in repair mode, a quiet digestive system, and a time of fasting? If this explanation of the advantages sounds a little like sleep mode, you're right! A good, normal night's sleep is a natural fasting period.

Fasting daily aids the body's alignment for sleep in many ways. Sleep disorders are often caused by eating in the evenings and having a body engaged in active digestion. Irrespective of the nutrient breakdown of the food we consume during those hours, studies show that reducing eating to 8- or 12-hour windows will help us maintain healthy body weight and prevent insulin resistance, high blood sugar, and diabetes.

The 24-hr circadian clocks, which have a strong effect on sleep, can be strengthened by time-restricted eating. A more synchronized circadian clock makes it easier to fall asleep, stay asleep, and wake up feeling refreshed daily. We all want the balance of continuity and quality in our sleep routines to help us feel and work at our best and protect the health over time and as we get older.

Fasting may affect sleep depending on when and how long it is done. According to some research, fasting regularly for a short period will help you sleep better. Fasting regularly was found to minimize nighttime awakenings and leg movements in one study (which can be strongly disruptive to sound sleep). Fasting has also been shown to minimize REM sleep in other studies.

Several patients who practice intermittent fasting say that it improves their sleep and also their waking performance. The majority find it relatively simple to adapt to a fasting state without experiencing heavy, disruptive hunger pangs. Even so, when fasting for a full day, people can feel more cravings and hunger. When you're hungry, falling asleep can be difficult. That's one aspect that might influence how fasting affects nighttime sleep.

Fasting's impact is likely to be determined by this individual's answer as well as the fast's details, such as length. More studies on the long-term effects of fasting on circadian rhythms, sleep, and other aspects of health are required. One of most manageable ways to integrate intermittent fasting into your everyday life is to set aside at least 12 hrs of eating-restricted time.

How to sleep well when fasting?

Pay attention to the body. We can learn a lot about the effect of diet on sleep from studies. However, no amount of analysis can provide us with all of the answers. The way we sleep in response to various eating plans varies from person to person. A 24-hour fast leaves you agitated at bedtime, whereas restricting eating after sunset may bring new soundness to sleep.

The sleep requirements are special, as are the reactions to diet and time-restricted feeding. To find the best sleep window, people often need to change the bedtimes and wake times. Similarly, to maintain an optimal eating and fasting routine, people often need to fine-tune the eating habits. Accepting and working through the individual reactions to fasting—physical, mental, and emotional reactions are all possible—is one way to make this eating technique work for you, not only during the day but also at night.

Keep yourself hydrated. When you're doing intermittent fasting or time-restricted eating, drinking plenty of water during the day will help with hunger, mental focus, mood, and energy. Staying hydrated would also result in a better night's sleep. Because of a dry mouth, nose, and throat, even mild dehydration may cause restless sleep and increase the risk of snoring.

Make the most of the meals. Intermittent fasting patients tell me how shocked they are by how easily their bodies respond to their eating occasional limits. Most people report that their hunger pangs pass easily and don't feel compelled to overeat or consume many unhealthy "treat" foods during their non-fasting periods.

If you eat a balanced diet during non-fasting hours, you'll reap the most benefits from fasting. Limit sugar and refined foods in favor of whole foods, high fiber, various vegetables and fruits, lean proteins such as chicken, and good fats from nuts and high-quality oils. These nutritious staples will provide your body with the nutrients it needs while also improving your energy levels during the day. You'll probably get a better night's sleep.

Be aware of the surroundings. Many patients have also been told that time-restricted feeding and intermittent fasting have helped them be more mindful. Mindfulness will also help you fast, overcome temporary cravings, and maintain a balanced diet. According to research, mindfulness will help in making better food choices. There's also a lot of proof that mindfulness activities help sleep better. It's not difficult to practice mindfulness: it's as simple as thinking, slow breathing or simple moving meditation.

6.6 Things to Do During Your Fasting Hours

1. Get flexible

Fasting makes exercise much more difficult, but there are other things you can engage in during Ramadan. Consider taking up yoga or Pilates. Both are excellent for maintaining mental and physical fitness and flexibility.

Doing a non-strengthening exercise when fasting should be a breeze if you eat nutritious meals in the evening and remain well hydrated. So, this Ramadan, try a new exercise like yoga or Pilates to kick-start your fitness routine and set yourself up for a versatile lifestyle!

2. Arrange a car boot sale.

Participating in or hosting your car boot sale can not only help you get rid of those unnecessary things clogging your wardrobe (come on, you know you'll never wear those shoes again); however, the money you raise will also go to a good cause (bonus points during Ramadan!) It's also a perfect way to forget about your empty stomach for a few days. Consider clothing, shoes, accessories, CDs, and other things you don't want and place a price on them. Once you've agreed on a time and place, enlist the fellow fasters' aid to support you or sell their things while having a good time with you!

3. Learn new skills

During Ramadan, participate in a course or a lecture series. Study a foreign language to boost your career opportunities and employability, or simply to connect more efficiently while on vacation. Or learn something new about a topic that has always sparked your interest. Whatever direction you choose, make sure you follow through and share with others. Why not bring along your fasting buddies while you're at it?

4. Take time to read

While we're on the topic of learning, why not read the book you've wanted to read for a while? Reading during your fasting hours is a perfect way to unwind and divert your attention away from hunger by transporting you to another world and time. You'll most likely take something away with you as well!

5. Help others

You cannot leave this one out because the spirit of Ramadan is focused on supporting and giving to others. You can help those in need in a variety of ways besides giving money. Even a smile, according to the Prophet (PBUH), is charity. Help a friend or family member with something they're having trouble with, whether it's their homework, a project they're working on, or just providing moral support. You may also support those who need food and shelter by volunteering at a homeless shelter. It doesn't matter what you do to make someone else happy!

6. Find a new hobby

Have you ever tried to learn a new hobby or talent but were unable to do so? What was it that held you back? Are you preoccupied? Is it the right time? What about studies? If you have the time and money, you will make good on your promise and learn the skill. Furthermore, educational institutions and workplaces are friendly and supportive to musical arts patrons, so you'd leave a mark.

7. Gardening as a hobby

Why not channel your energy into something useful? Learn to write, gardening, and make origami. Each of these activities is a combination of mental and physical exercises that assist in the relaxation of both the mind and body. You won't note the passage of time until you've submerged yourself in either one.

8. Clear the backlog

When you're engrossed in a good book or a good TV show, time flies. This summer is jam-packed with completely fantastic shows that will make time fly by.

6.7 Use of Detoxifying and Cleansing Smoothies

Detoxification (detox) diets have never been more common. These diets help to purify your blood and rid your body of dangerous toxins. However, it's unclear how they do it, what compounds they're going to get rid of, and if they work. It is a comprehensive look at detox diets and potential health impacts.

What Is a Detox?

Detox diets are usually short-term dietary treatments that aim to rid the body of toxins.

A standard detox diet includes a fasting time followed by a strict diet of vegetables, fruit, fruit juices, and water. Sometimes a detox also includes herbs, supplements, teas, and colon cleanse or enemas.

It is claimed that it will:

- Fasting allows the organs to rest.
- Toxins can be removed faster if the liver is stimulated.
- Urine, feces, and sweat can aid toxin removal.
- Improve the circulation.
- Give your body some healthy nutrients.

Detox treatments are often prescribed due to possible exposure to harmful chemicals in the atmosphere or the diet. Pollutants, heavy metals, synthetic chemicals, and other harmful compounds are among them.

Obesity, autoimmune diseases, digestive issues, bloating, inflammation, chronic fatigue, and allergies are among the health conditions these diets are said to help.

Human research on detox diets, on the other hand, is limited, and the few studies that do exist are severely flawed.

Detoxes are short-term treatments that help the body rid itself of toxins. They're said to help with many health issues.

The Most Common Detox Methods

A detox diet can be achieved in many ways, from full starvation to easy food modifications. At least one of the following is used in most detox diets:

- 1–3 days of fasting
- Fresh vegetable and fruit juices, water, smoothies, and tea are all good options.
- Only drinking certain liquids, such as salted water or lemon juice.
- Foods rich in heavy metals, allergens, and contaminants should be avoided.
- Taking herbal or nutritional supplements.
- All allergenic foods should be avoided for a while before being progressively reintroduced.
- Laxatives, enemas, or colon cleanses are all options.
- Exercising daily.
- Eliminating cigarettes, coffee, alcohol, and refined sugar.

The intensity and length of detox diets vary. Detoxes come in a variety of ways. Fasting, consuming specific foods, avoiding harmful ingredients, or taking supplements.

Which Toxins Are Removed?

Detox diets often indicate which toxins they are trying to eliminate. The mechanisms that enable them to function are also unknown.

Detox diets, in reality, provide little or no evidence of removing toxins from the body.

Furthermore, the feces, liver, sweat, and urine are all capable of cleaning the body. Toxic substances are made harmless by your liver, which means that they are expelled from your body.

Despite this, certain chemicals, such as phthalates, persistent organic pollutants (POPs), heavy metals, and bisphenol A (BPA), can be difficult to extract using these techniques.

These appear to collect in fat tissue or blood, and flushing them out can take a long time — even years.

Today, however, these compounds are usually excluded from or restricted in commercial products.

Overall, there is no proof that detox diets help in the removal of any of the compounds.

What Is the Effectiveness of These Diets?

During and after detox diets, some people feel more concentrated and energetic.

However, your better health may be simply a result of removing alcohol, processed foods, and other harmful substances from your diet.

It's also possible that you're getting minerals and vitamins that you didn't have before.

However, several people report feeling severely sick during the detox process.

Effects on Weight Loss

Only a few research studies have looked at the effects of detox diets on weight loss. Although some people may lose so much weight quickly, this effect seems to be due to fluid and carbohydrate loss rather than fat loss. When you stop doing the cleanse, you normally gain weight easily.

Lemon detox diet restricts you to a combination of palm syrups or organic maple & lemon juice for 7 days. It was examined in overweight Korean women.

This diet decreases body weight, body fat percentage, BMI, waist circumference, waist-to-hip ratio, insulin resistance, inflammation markers, and circulating leptin levels significantly.

A detox diet that requires extreme calorie restriction will almost certainly result in weight loss and changes in metabolic health, but it is unlikely to help you maintain your weight loss over time.

Stress, Detox Diets, and Short-Term Fasting

Several detox diets have been shown to have similar effects to short-term or intermittent fasting. In certain people, fasting for a short period may increase disease markers such as insulin and leptin sensitivity.

These results, however, do not extend to everyone. A 48-hour fast and 3 weeks of decreased calorie intake have increased stress hormone levels in women studies. Furthermore, since they include fighting temptations and experiencing intense hunger, extreme diets can be a traumatic experience.

Detox diets can help with weight loss in the short term, but more research is required. Some detox diets are similar to intermittent fasting, which may boost some health biomarkers.

Potential Benefits

Several aspects of detox diets could be beneficial to your health, including:

- Avoiding POPs and heavy metals in your diet
- Excessive fat loss
- Sweating and exercising regularly
- Consumption of whole, nutritious, and healthful foods
- Processed foods should be avoided.
- Green tea and water are healthy for you.
- Relaxing, limiting stress, and getting enough sleep are all necessary.

Whether or not you're on a detox diet, following these guidelines has been linked to better health.

Detox diets can benefit your health in several ways. Avoiding environmental toxins, drinking plenty of water, eating nutritious foods, limiting stress, exercising, and relaxing are just a few of them.

Chapter No 7: Exercise Plan during Intermittent Fasting

Get-Fit Ideas for Women over 50 are as follows:

- Staying Fit as you age

- Make exercise a part of the Daily Routine

It's fantastic if you were physically fit before the age of 50. However, if you haven't been exercising regularly, it isn't too late to begin.

Hot flashes, joint pain, and sleep issues are symptoms of menopause that can benefit from physical activity. Exercise will also help you prevent heart disease, diabetes, and osteoporosis. It also helps in weight loss and the reduction of belly fat. Exercise has such powerful effects that it influences each physiological function in the body for good.

7.1 Keeping Fit as You Get Older

Many age issues are related to an inactive lifestyle. While the chronological age may be above 50, the biological age can be below 40 if you stick to a regular exercise routine. Consult your doctor before beginning, particularly if you have any heart disease risk factors (high blood pressure, smoking, diabetes, high cholesterol, or family history). Then it's time to get going.

The following information must be included in a detailed fitness program:

- Aerobic exercise: Try walking, swimming, jogging, or dancing as a form of exercise. Aerobic exercise works your body's large muscles, which benefits the cardiovascular system and the weight. Work your way up to 20 or more mins per session, three or four days a week. Please ensure you can pass the "talk test," which requires you to exercise at a speed that allows you to converse.

- Strength training: Hand weights lifting strengthens your strength and balance, keeps your bones healthy, decreases your risk of back injury, and strengthens your muscles. Start with an eight-repetition of hand weight which you can comfortably handle. Gradually increase the number of reps until you can perform 12 in a row.

- Stretching: Stretching exercises help maintain range of motion and flexibility in joints. They also help to avoid injuries and muscle soreness. Pilates and yoga are excellent stretching exercises that strengthen the core body and improve stability.

- Include exercise in your everyday routine.

- Every little bit of movement makes a difference. If you don't have time for a daily workout, find other ways to stay healthy. According to the study, all of the extra actions you take throughout the day contribute to major health benefits. Here are some tips to help you get back on your feet:

- Buy a dog and take it for regular walks.

- Instead of taking the elevator, take the stairs. Don't yell at your family from the top of the stairs; instead, go up.

- Rather than sending texts, get up and chat with colleagues. Are you having a meeting with any work colleague? Make it a walking meeting by taking it outside.

- When you have the opportunity, take a quick walk. Often wear or carry comfortable shoes so that the feet can be the primary mode of transportation.

- Choose a sport, activity, or game that you enjoy. If you like what you're doing, you'll be more motivated to exercise.

7.2 Strength Training Moves for Women Over 50

Life moves too quickly. You can realize as you get older how important it is to make the most of every day. So, how to delay the onset of aging? Although we cannot turn back the time, we can try to turn back the bodies' years by exercising.

Exercise has been shown to slow down the physical aging clock in studies. Yes, working out will help you stay young.

Although aerobic exercises like walking, jogging, or biking are beneficial for heart and lung health, strength training keeps the body looking stronger, younger, and more functional with each passing year.

This strength-training routine will assist you in remaining lively and self-sufficient for several more years.

Benefits of Strength Training After 50

Everyone benefits from strength training, but after the age of 50, it becomes much more necessary. It becomes less about having big biceps or flat abs and more about maintaining a solid, balanced body that is less prone to injury and illness.

"Sedentary adults may experience as much as a 30 percent to 40 percent loss of muscular strength because of reduced levels of muscle mass between the ages of 30 and 80," according to the American Council on Exercise.

After 50, strength training benefits the body in the following ways:

Builds bone density: Every year, countless older people are admitted to hospitals due to unexpected falls. An 8-year-old has a cast on his arm and returns to play in 8 weeks. An 80-year-old isn't in such good shape. Broken bones can have far-reaching effects. Physical training can be helpful.

No, this does not imply that you can turn into the Hulk. It signifies that you are a solid, powerful individual capable of lifting your groceries, pushing your lawnmower, and picking yourselves up if you fall.

Reduces body fat: Having too much body fat is unhealthy at any age. Maintaining a healthy weight is critical, especially when it comes to avoiding many diseases that affect the elderly.

Improves mental health: As people age, they are more likely to experience depression and, to most, a lack of self-confidence. Strength training has been shown to enhance general self-efficacy and can even help you prevent depression.

Reduces the risk of chronic illness: Strength training is recommended by the Centers for Disease Control and Prevention (CDC) for many older adults to help relieve the effects of chronic conditions such as diabetes, osteoporosis, back pain, obesity, arthritis, and depression.

Power training is a successful investment. You will see significant improvements in your body's age in just 20 to 30 mins a day. So let's get this started. The following workout will provide you with ten incredible exercises that females over 50 can use in their workouts.

Single-leg moves and stability ball moves will be used in some exercises. These were included to aid in the improvement of balance and coordination, which both worsen with age. A stability ball and a pair of 3 to 8 lbs hand weights (move up to heavier weights when you get stronger) are needed.

You can do the exercises on the ground or a bench if you don't have a ball. Perform 8 -12 repetitions of each exercise below, pausing for 30 to 60 seconds between sets. Slowly work your way through each workout, focusing on correct shape and breathing.

Also, having a team to exercise with is often beneficial, so look for nearby fitness classes or rally your mates. Furthermore, if you have access to a fitness specialist, even if only for one session, they will help you learn proper form and teach you how to move correctly for your body. Take advantage of the new fountain of youth.

1. Forearm Plank

Start by lying on the ground with the forearms flat on the ground and the elbows directly under the shoulders.

Lift your body off the floor by engaging your core and holding the forearms on the floor and the body in a straight line from head to feet. Maintain abdominal engagement and stop causing the hips to rise or fall. Keep for 30 seconds instead of 8 to 12 reps. Place the knees on the ground if it hurts the low back or it becomes too difficult.

Shoulders and core are the main targets.

2. Modified Push-Up

Begin on a mat, kneeling with hands under shoulders and knees behind the hips to create an angled and long back.

To lower the chest toward the floor, tuck the toes under, tighten the abdominals, and bend the elbows. Maintain a long neck by holding your gaze in front of the fingertips. Return the chest to the starting position.

Shoulders, arms, and core are the primary targets.

3. Basic Squat

Standing tall with the feet hip-distance apart is a good place to start. Y our hips, knees, and toes should face forward. (Hold dumbbells in the hands to make it difficult). As if you were going to lean back into a chair, bend your knees and stretch your buttocks backward. Make sure your knees are behind the toes, and the weight is balanced by your feet. Return to your feet and repeat the process.

Gluteus Maximus, quadriceps Maximus, and hamstrings Maximus targeted.

4. Stability Ball Chest Fly

Place both shoulder blades and head on top of the ball, with the rest of the body in a tabletop position, while holding a pair of dumbbells close to the stomach. The feet should be hip-distance apart. Raise dumbbells together, palms facing in and straight above the chest. Slowly lower your arms out to the side, keeping your elbows slightly bent, until your elbows are around chest level. Squeeze your chest and pull both your hands back at the top.

Chest, glutes, back, and core are the muscles targeted.

5. Stability Ball Triceps Kick Back

Place your chest on the ball, arms crossed alongside the ball, and legs extended out towards the floor behind you while holding dumbbells. Maintain a straight line between your head and your spine. (If you don't have a ball, lie down on your stomach on a bench or stand with your feet staggered and your body hinged forward.) To begin, bring your elbow up to a 90-degree angle. Squeeze triceps when pressing dumbbells back to lengthen muscles. Return the dumbbells to their starting spot.

The triceps and core are the muscles targeted.

6. Shoulder Overhead Press

Start with your feet hip-width apart. Bring your elbows out to the side to form a goal post with your arms, dumbbells to the side of your back, and abs strong. Slowly raise dumbbells until arms are straight. Return to the starting point slowly and steadily. This exercise can also be done sitting in a chair or on a stability ball with your feet spread wide if needed.

Shoulders, biceps, and back are the main targets.

7. Overhead Pull with a Stability Ball

Place your shoulder blades and head on top of the ball, with the rest of your body in a tabletop position, while holding a pair of dumbbells close to your stomach. The distance between your feet should be hip-width apart. Raise dumbbells straight above the chest, palms facing in, and slowly lower arms behind the back of the head, holding the elbows just slightly bent.

Move arms to the starting position just above the chest while squeezing your lats.

Back and core are the primary targets.

8. Stability Leg Lift on the Ball Side

Kneel with the ball to the right side and begin. Allow your right side to lean on the ball and wrap the right arm around it. Extend the left leg to the side. The right leg should be bent on the floor at all times. Slowly lift and lower the left leg eight to twelve times before switching sides.

Legs and core are the primary targets.

9. Hamstring Bridge with a Single Leg

Lie on your back with your knees bent and your feet flat on the meat. In a bridge position, squeeze glutes and raise hips off the mat. Lower and raise the hips for 10-12 reps, then switch sides.

Hamstrings, glutes, and quadriceps are the muscles targeted.

10. Bird Dog

Kneel on all fours on the mat. Move one arm behind you, pull in your abs, and stretch the opposite leg behind you.

Repeat 8–12 times on each side, then switch sides.

7.3 Best Types of Exercise for Older Women

Integrate these top fitness strategies into the training plan to stay strong, stay healthy, and maintain your freedom.

The best workout for senior citizens. The best workout for you, regardless of your age, is one you like most. So After all, how long will you stick with a workout if you don't like it?

Even so, it's important to remember what you may want and have to be out of the workout while trying any of the countless styles of exercise available. According to Barbara Bergin, the M.D., who is orthopedic doctor in Austin, Texas, this is bound to improve over time. She states that improving the quality of the life outside of the gym should be a top priority for older adults.

To do so, concentrate on exercises that will help you gain stamina, agility, and balance. It's also important to think about what each fitness choice needs. Are the bones able to withstand high-impact activities like running & jumping? Is the balance in the right place for the fall-free rides of bikes ? How much more time do you have to invest at the gym regularly?

best exercise for older people are listed below, according to experts. Before starting a new exercise program, always consult your doctor, particularly if you've chronic illness, balance problems, or even injuries. good news is that as long as your doctor hasn't told you otherwise, you can do anything you want—they're all great.

1. Swimming

Swimming is known as "the world's perfect workout" for a reason. Whether you're taking water aerobics, doing the breaststroke, or playing the MarcoPolo with kids, getting in the swimming pool is a good method to increase cardiovascular fitness and also strengthen the muscles.

It accomplishes all of this with minimal stress upon the joints and bones, which is huge advantage for women and men with osteoporosis or arthritis. As if it wasn't enough, a 2012 report published in Journal of the Aging Science claims that swimming as an exercise can help the older people retain their mental sharpness as well as their physical ability.

2. Yoga

According to David Kruse, the M.D., sports medicine professional at Hoag Orthopedics Institute in California, yoga helps develop aerobic fitness, muscle strength, total-body mobility, and core stability —all of which are vital for older adults.

Although yoga's low-impact & gentle on the joints, it is also weight-bearing, which means you must support your body's weight at all times. Not only the muscles but the bones will also benefit from this.

If you're new to yoga, participate in an introductory class to learn the basics. SilverSneakers Yoga is designed for seniors and includes a chair so that you can do poses while sitting or standing. Restorative yoga, hatha yoga, and Iyengar yoga are all excellent choices. Before you begin, discuss any physical limitations with your teacher.

3. Pilates

Pilates, just like yoga, is famous for being a low-impact method of strength, but its emphasis on the core stability which makes it particularly beneficial to seniors, according to Dr. Shin. Pilates involvement increases the balance in the older adults.

Many gyms have Pilates classes for beginners, particularly useful for those participating in classes which use the "reformer," a resistance-training system with bars, springs, and belts. You can also try this at-home Pilates exercise to strengthen the core.

4. Bodyweight Exercises

According to a study published in the journal Age and Ageing, one in every 3 older people suffers from extreme muscle loss. Meanwhile, Harvard research indicates that strength exercise is much time-effective than aerobic exercise in reducing age-related abdominal fat, a proxy for overall health.

Dr. Shin says that you don't need to just bench press a lot of weight in order to keep the muscles balanced and avoid fat expansion over time. In reality, she points out that for older people, starting small is much better. Chair squats, wall pushups, stair climbing, and single-leg stands are excellent bodyweight exercises for keeping the body healthy and ready for daily activities.

All you need to learn about strength training is right here. Are you ready to give it a shot? Begin by squatting in a chair.

5. Workouts with Resistance Bands

Resistance bands are certainly available at the gym, but these cheap & beginner-friendly fitness tools are also ideal for workouts at-home.

Furthermore, bands will help you to challenge the muscles in the ways that equipment-free training may not do so. Rows, as well as other pulling motions, for example, are important for strengthening the back & improving the posture—but they're difficult to do even if you don't have any workout equipment on the hand.

6. Walking

If you don't have time to do structured workout, Dr. Shin says you probably have enough time to place 1 foot in the front of other to go where you have to. And on days that they don't "rock out," she advises that most people walk 10 thousand steps a day. People who raised their exercise levels to ten thousand steps a day were about 46 % less likely to be dying in 10 years than those who remained sedentary (according to research published in PLOS One).

10 thousand might not be the correct exact amount for certain older adults or people with chronic conditions. However, the truth remains that walking is fantastic, free exercise that can significantly improve your fitness.

7. Cycling

Cycling, one more low-impact type of exercise, is suitable for the ones who'd want to strengthen their legs but can't run or participate in other high-impact sports because of osteoporosis or the joint problems, according to Dr. Shin. Cycling helps enhance metabolic health, cardiovascular health, & cognitive performances in adults over 70, according to a 2017 study published in the European Review of Aging and Physical Activity.

If you live near a bike path, consider organizing monthly rides of bike with friends or family. If you don't have access to the trails or the weather isn't cooperating, indoor cycling is a perfect alternative. You also don't have to think about falling or wearing a helmet while riding a stationary bike.

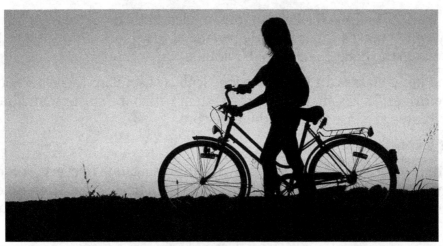

8. Aerobic and Strength Training

If you've ever attended a SilverSneakers class, you know that group workout isn't just a great way to work up a sweat. Along the way, you'll have a lot of fun and meet new people, both of which are crucial for making workouts a habit. According to a 2017 study published in BMC Public Health, group exercise's social side improves activity levels in older people over time.

9. Personal Training

Working with a personal trainer is a fantastic way to get fit and have fun if you want more attention and instruction than group classes would offer. Many have one-on-one and small-group workouts, with the latter consisting of you and one or three mates doing the same exercise with the trainer. Use one-on-one sessions; you get started with a plan that you can proceed on your own or go the small-group route to save money.

Regardless of which choice you select, the trainer will help you learn proper form and build a strong foundation of exercise experience that you will use for years to come. Also, the workouts will most likely include a variety of exercises.

Chapter No 8: FAQs about Intermittent Fasting

8.1. What Is Intermittent Fasting, and How Is the Diet Different From Starvation?

According to Johns Hopkins Medicine, Intermittent Fasting is a form of eating that involves switching between fasting (or a substantial reduction in calorie intake) and eating at particular times. It differs from several other diets in that it does not require the consumption of particular foods. It's also not about deprivation with IF. Rather, it entails taking your meals at specific times and fast for the remainder of the day and night.

8.2. What Is the History of Intermittent Fasting (and Fasting in General)?

According to a report published in the Journal of the Academy of Nutrition and Dietetics in August 2015, fasting has been around since ancient times and is primarily practiced within religions. However, the current version of IF emerged in the last 8 years or so. According to Harvard Health, when the documentary Eat, Quick, and Live Longer aired in 2012, IF became more famous. According to the Journal of the Academy of Nutrition and Dietetics research, many books on the subject were also released around that time, including 2013's The Quick Diet, which added to the buzz. Then came the study. "Rough research has shown the amazing advantages of intermittent fasting over the past five years," says Sara Gottfried, MD, author of Brain-Body Diet, based in Berkeley, California.

8.3. How Does Intermittent Fasting Work?

According to Harvard Health, there are few different IF. Still, each one follows the basic principle of designating a certain amount of time during the week for eating and a certain period during the week when drink and food should be restricted (or extremely limited).

8.4. What Are the Different Types of Intermittent Fasting?

The most popular are:

- 16:8: This approach calls for fasting for 16 hours and feeding for 8 hours during the day. The majority of people who follow this practice miss breakfast and feed between 11 a.m. to 7 p.m. or noon to 8 p.m. Fasting continues through the night and into the morning. This method is known as "time-restricted feeding," according to Dr. Lowden.

- Fasting on alternate days: According to a report published in Translational Research in October 2014, this means restricting your calories to 25% of your normal calorie intake accompanied by a regular eating day. For example, on Mondays, Wednesdays, and Fridays, you could restrict calories heavily but eat regularly on the other days.

- 5:2 Fasting: On the 2 non consecutive "fasting" times of the week, a very small number of calories (approximately 400 to 500 calories) is permitted. According to Harvard, the other five days have no dietary restrictions.

8.5. Can Intermittent Fasting Help You Lose Weight?

Dr. Gottfried says, "Intermittent Fasting gets lots of press as a weight-loss tool, and I suggest it in my practice for weight loss and weight control." According to Harvard Health, it's related to weight loss as not eating in between meals causes the body to depend on fat deposited in cells for energy. Insulin levels fall as the body burns fat in this process.

But, according to Lowden, what it boils down to is calorie restriction. "Overall, as opposed to eating all day, people prefer to consume fewer calories in a shorter window of time, which contributes to losing weight," she says. A study of 23 obese adults published in June 2018 in Nutrition and Healthy Aging found that when they followed the 16:8 approach to IF, they consumed about 300 fewer calories per day.

According to a report published in December 2018 in BMC Public Health, versions of IF that limit eating after a certain period, such as 7 p.m., help prevent nighttime eating, and linked to metabolic syndrome and obesity.

However, some critics argue that the amount of weight loss achieved by IF is comparable to that achieved by other calorie-restrictive diets. According to a report published in the American Journal of Clinical Nutrition in November 2018, a diet that reduced calories by 20% resulted in comparable weight loss after one year as the 5:2 variant of IF. Still, if you find it easier to adhere to than other diets, IF could be a good choice.

8.6. What Are the Benefits of Intermittent Fasting?

Here are some of the proposed benefits of IF:

- Boost your weight loss efforts. The majority of research on IF has supported its contribution to weight loss, according to a study released in Current Obesity Reports in June 2018. The results indicate that it may result in a 5 to 9.9% loss of body weight. According to a 2018 study released in Nutrition and Healthy Aging, alternate fasting can achieve greater weight loss than time-restricted eating. Still, alternate-day fasting may be more difficult to maintain than time-restricted eating. Finally, more research is required to see if Intermittent Fasting can lead to actual, long-term weight loss.

- Extending your life Calorie restriction can delay aging, according to a study released in Cell in December 2014. However, the research was conducted on livestock, and the results have yet to be replicated in humans.

- Insulin resistance is reduced. According to a study published in Frontiers of Medicine in February 2014, insulin resistance is a characteristic of type 2 diabetes, and being overweight raises the risk of developing it. According to a study released in Nutrients in April 2019, IF can help with insulin resistance by lowering total calorie consumption.

- Improved cardiovascular wellbeing According to a study, Intermittent Fasting helped study women lose weight, fat, and cholesterol levels, leading experts to believe that eating this way might reduce their risk of coronary artery disease.

- Enhance metabolic functions Lowden says, "What we do know is that a lot of such metabolic parameters lead to weight loss in general." "You'll have reduced visceral (belly) fat, reduced fasting blood sugars, reduced triglycerides, blood sugar, and all those things no matter how you lose weight." It has been seen in a few animal experiments, according to Lowden, but "a lot of the stuff you'd physiologically anticipate from a longer quick time isn't panning out in population studies."

8.7. Who Shouldn't Try Intermittent Fasting, Because of Safety Concerns?

The following types of people should avoid IF:

- Diabetic people (not before asking a doctor). According to a study conducted in August 2019 in Nutrients, while IF can increase insulin sensitivity and help patients with diabetes (type 2), it can also be dangerous for people taking diabetes drugs that cause hypoglycemia (low blood sugar), such as insulin. As a result, people with diabetes (type 1) who depend on insulin should avoid Intermittent Fasting.

- People who suffer from other chronic illnesses. According to the 2019 Nutrients review, little is known about how fasting affects many chronic diseases, women with diabetes, but negative side effects, including nausea and dizziness, could be more pronounced for these individuals. According to Lowden, when you have medical problems that may be exacerbated by not eating properly, you must be cautious.

- People who are overweight. According to a study released in Nutrients in March 2019, those with a BMI of less than 18.5 are not recommended to try weight-loss diets that include IF.

- People who are either suffering from or have a history of eating disorders. According to the Harvard School of Public Health, IF can promote an unhealthy relationship with food. Some people could be tempted to be using the end of the fast as an excuse to cheat on unhealthy foods, according to a study reported in Current Obesity in June 2019.

- Senior citizens. According to a Nutrients report published in March 2019, fasting can increase the risk of stroke, cardiovascular disease, and arrhythmia in the elderly.

- Women who are expecting a child or who are breastfeeding. According to the Mayo Clinic, breastfeeding isn't the best time to fast or cut calories, according to the same report, since women need an additional 300 to 500 calories a day to maintain milk production and energy levels.

- According to Harvard Health, people who need to take medicine with food must eat regularly to avoid missing a dose.

- According to Johns Hopkins, everybody should consult a doctor before beginning a fast, whether they have any of the conditions mentioned above.

8.8. Is It Good or Bad to Exercise While Intermittent Fasting?

One theory, according to Harvard, is that exercising when fasted will help burn fat. Lowden states that the body requires sugar or other kinds of energy to exercise effectively. Sugar molecules that are processed as glycogen in the liver provide the energy in most cases. "If you start exercising, you're more likely to reduce those stores, and your body will have no choice but to go through an anaerobic breakdown to provide you with the energy you require," she explains. The body is forced to burn off another energy source: fat, instead of sugars that aren't available.

However, you can lack the energy to work out as regularly as you usually would. "It's much easier to achieve peak efficiency or even feel healthy when exercising if you feed," Lowden says.

8.9. What's the Best Way to Manage Hunger While Fasting?

You'll probably feel hungry as the body transitions to IF, but Gottfried promises that it will. "It gets easier," she says, based on her own experience and input from her patients. According to a Harvard University study, intermittent Fasting (IF) does not increase overall appetite. The 16:8 diet (or any variant thereof), according to Gottfried, appears to be the simplest for several people to incorporate into their lifestyles without feeling hungry.

8.10. What Side Effects Can I Expect on an Intermittent Fasting Diet?

Transitioning to this way of eating is difficult for many people. According to a study published in April 2019 in Nutrients, IF can cause migraines, dizziness, nausea, and insomnia. It can also make people feel hungry and tired during the day, limiting their activity.

According to the same Nutrients research, some women could stop menstruating because of calorie restriction. According to the Mayo Clinic, if you miss 3 periods in a row, you should see a doctor.

8.11. What Is the Best Way to Get Started on a Fasting Diet?

Before getting into IF, think about your health goals and take the following steps:

Consult your primary care physician. He or she will tell you if this diet plan is good for your health. "It's important to speak with healthcare practitioners if you have concerns about what's best for you," Lowden advises. "Everyone is different, and depending on the situation, the doctor may have ideas for what you do and avoid."

Select the most appropriate form of IF for you. If you often socialize late at night, for example, 5:2 is likely to be a better option than 16:8. If you plan to try 16:8, Gottfried recommends starting slowly. "I suggest beginning slowly and gradually increasing your fasting time and eating window, starting with a 12-hour fast and a 12-hour eating window, then moving up to a 14-hour fast and a 10-hour eating window, and finally to 16:8," she says, and also emphasizes the importance of remembering that the eating and fasting windows are flexible. "Some people tend to eat at 10 a.m. then stop at 6 p.m.; many prefer to eat at noon and stop at 8 p.m.," she explains. "Find something that fits you."

Please ensure you have plenty of water on hand. According to the 2019 Nutrients report, drinking lots of water throughout the day can help you avoid dehydration and substitute fluids that you would usually get from food.

Physical activity should be restricted. Limiting your behaviors during the fasting windows is also a good idea, according to Gottfried, before you know how the body will respond.

8.12. What Is the Best Way to Break a Fast and Begin Eating Again?

Don't use the end of the fast as an opportunity to binge on unhealthy foods; this could hinder the diet's chances of success. "Whether it's a time-restricted feeding or regular overnight fast, the concepts of healthy eating and ending a fast are the same," Lowden says. Break your fast with a nutritious, well-balanced meal rich in lean proteins, complex carbohydrates, and good fats.

Protein should be given special attention, particularly if you already have diabetes. "We always recommend eating a type of protein with every meal, especially when you're breaking a fast, to control normal sugar levels and prevent worsening insulin resistance," Lowden says. According to Diabetes.co.uk, protein does not break down into glucose as quickly as carbohydrates, so it has a gradual, less rapid effect on blood sugar levels.

Breaking your fast with a good source of carbs, according to Gottfried, will help to restore reduced glycogen levels. She suggests a Mediterranean-style meal consisting of 40% carbohydrates, 30% protein, and 30% fat.

Lowden also claims that the order in which you break your fast will make a difference. "Studies show that people who consume their calories later in the day, even though they consume the same amount of calories, weigh more than people who consume their calories early in the day," Lowden says. According to a study released in Nutrients in April 2015, sleep-deprived women with late sleep patterns are more likely to gain weight because foods consumed at night are higher in fat than foods eaten early in the day. Take this into account when deciding on your eating window.

8.13. How Does Intermittent Fasting Work?

Intermittent fasting functions similarly to a low-carb diet. When you extend the time b/w meals, your body is forced to depend on stored energy. You can continue to develop ketones as a by-product of fat burning, depending on what you eat between fasts and how long you go between eating periods. When you go more than a few hours without feeding, the blood insulin levels drop, which is a proven advantage of IF. It helps your body to burn fat that has been stored and may increase insulin sensitivity.

8.14. What is the Science behind Intermittent Fast?

Although there is evidence that Intermittent Fasting (IF) can be effective, many studies use different fasting approaches, making the study difficult to review. Some studies indicate that eating 14:10 is beneficial, whereas others look at the advantages of fasting on alternating days. One thing to keep in mind is that clinical trials using IF are usually shorter than two years, so this strategy's long-term viability is still unknown. Furthermore, it is unclear if intermittent fasting advantages are derived directly from fasting or indirectly by weight loss.

8.15. What are the Advantages of Intermittent Fasting?

Intermittent fasting appears to be beneficial for weight loss and maintenance and enhances digestive function, metabolic health, and circadian rhythm. According to other studies, IF helps people lose weight, maintain stable blood glucose levels, and control inflammation by reducing caloric intake. Some researchers believe that Intermittent Fasting can help support cognitive functions and even break food addiction, resulting in weight loss.

8.16. What are the Popular Types of Intermittent Fasting?

There are several different forms of IF, but they can be divided into three categories.

- Time-restricted eating– This form of intermittent fasting divides the 24-hour day into fast and feeding windows. 12:12, 16:8, and 20:4 are examples of common time-restricted eating plans.

- Alternate-Day Fasting – While it might sound like you should fast any other day, this is a word that refers to a practice of eating normally one day and consuming very few calories the next (around 500 calories). The 5:2 method of fasting on alternative-day includes eating normally for five days and fasting or eating a very low-calorie diet for the remaining two days of week.

- Longer fasts – When people become more familiar with IF, they can begin to read about fasts lasting 24 hours or more. We don't usually advise people to follow this method because eating low carb is a healthy way of eating that offers a full nutritional profile without requiring you to go without food for days on end. Anyone considering a longer fast should speak with a healthcare provider who specializes in this form of fasting.

8.17. How Long Should I Fast?

If you want to try intermittent fasting, we recommend beginning with a 14:10 or 16:8 schedule. It allows you to gradually train your body to rely on its energy reserves without overtaxing it right away. Even these short fasts are effective for weight loss and improving metabolic health markers. We recommend using Intermittent Fasting (IF) to get back on track rather than a permanent diet.

8.18. When Should I Fast?

When you know you have a lot of blood sugar & insulin, getting rid of Intermittent Fasting is possibly the best option. It could be after the holidays or after a week or 2 if you haven't been consuming low carb for a while.

After dinner, it is recommended to begin with a 16-hour easy. Dinner should be finished between 6-7 p.m. if possible. On Monday, and your next meal will not be until 10-11 a.m. this coming Tuesday. It is suggested to stay hydrated and eating enough electrolytes during your fasting time.

You can follow your chosen fasting method for almost as long as you want, whether it's one day or a year. Some people fast because they are bloated or have eaten too much the previous night, while others fast as a way of life. Pay close attention to how you're feeling and tailor it to your preferences.

8.19. What Should I Eat When I'm Not Fasting

The majority of IF research does not have specific recommendations about what to consume during the feeding window. However, regardless of the type of fasting you want, make sure you're getting enough good calories during the feeding window. Avoid sugar and processed carbohydrates in favor of healthier foods, including healthy fats, fiber-rich carbs, and protein (roughly 12-18 ounces per day).

Since some of the fasting's benefits come from lowering insulin output, it's become fashionable to combine it with a low-carb or keto diet. When you're not fasting, eat high-quality foods.

8.20. What Should I Eat to Break My Fast?

When you're able to eat again after a short fast, try not to lose any of the metabolic advantages you've acquired during your fast. It means avoiding high-glycemic foods like junk food and sugar and replacing them with low-glycemic foods like cooked vegetables, fruit, or poultry/fish. If you've been fasting for a while, it's a good idea to ease your digestive system back into action with something simple to digest like a smoothie or broth/soup.

8.21. What are the Side Effects of Intermittent Fasting?

When you start IF, the decrease in insulin levels & carb intake, similar to when you start a keto diet, can cause water & electrolyte loss. Some people experience headaches, flu-like symptoms, or low blood pressure/dizziness due to this. If you are not adjusted to IF or are using blood sugar lowering medications, you can experience low blood sugar levels. Pay close attention to how you're feeling, and don't be afraid to break the fast early if you're feeling under the weather.

It's important to remember that IF isn't for everybody. If you have diabetes, you can have your medicine closely monitored by a doctor because you are at risk of being hypoglycemic, which can be deadly. Anyone who has suffered from an eating problem, has preexisting conditions, is under 18, or is pregnant, or breastfeeding should avoid Intermittent Fasting.

Consult your doctor/healthcare provider before beginning any new workout routine to see if intermittent fasting is good for you.

8.22. How Do I Combine Fasting with Atkins 20?

It is not recommended to combine these two methods. If you want to combine the two, begin your low-carb diet 2–3 weeks before fasting so that the body can adjust safely and fully.

Intermittent fasting should be combined with an Atkins 100-style diet, which allows for more fiber-rich carbs each day. It will help to alleviate some of the tension that comes with strict carbohydrate restriction and Intermittent Fasting. Atkins 100 is also more in line with studies that have combined low-carb feeding with fasting.

8.23. Can I Exercise During the Fasting Period?

Some people experience dizziness or low blood pressure/blood sugar while fasting. Starting with gentle exercise and paying attention to how you feel throughout your workouts is a good idea.

8.24. Is there a best time (of the day) to fast?

According to current human research, there is no clarity about the best meal timing for people practicing intermittent fasting. As the day goes on, you become more insulin resistant or less able to clear blood sugar levels and transport it to where it requires to go in the body. As a result, it's probably better to eat most of the calories earlier during the day and begin your fasting window some hours before bedtime.

Dr. Krista Varady advises, "Your body can't cope with nutrients (glucose) as effectively later in the day, so you may as well give the body a break from glucose then." "Your body is loaded and ready to cope with an influx of nutrients early in the day."

If you follow an alternate-day fasting schedule and eat less than 500 calories on the fast days, you can consume these calories all at once or spread them out over three small meals during the day. Allowing for flexibility in meal timing on quick days can help you stick to your fasting routine in the long run.

8.25. Is there a best way to break my fast?

Different forms of post-fast foods on metabolic health have yet to be thoroughly tested in scientific research studies.

Following a high-carbohydrate post-fast meal, a small number of studies suggest that certain people will experience an immediate blood sugar spike associated with insulin resistance. On the other hand, acute postprandial insulin resistance could be more common in people who aren't used to fasting for long periods (16-24 hours). If you're new to fasting, start by breaking your fasts with meals that are low in glycemic index and high in fiber and plant fats (avocado, olives, seeds, nuts, coconut, etc.) After a few months of intermittent fasting, the body is likely to have various metabolic reactions to an excess of nutrients after the fast. Over time, IF usually results in lower blood glucose levels and increased insulin sensitivity.

8.26. Is it okay to exercise while fasting?

Yes. Compared to either workout or fasting alone, combining fast with endurance training can produce superior improvements in weight, body composition, and lipid indications of heart disease risk.

Contrary to common opinion, exercising on alternating fast days or during fasts of less than 24 hours is healthy. In reality, in IF studies, participants often report feeling more energized on days when they fast or consume less than 500 calories.

"You can observe reductions in energy or attention levels in the 10 days of an alternate day of fasting practice," Dr. Krista Varady says. "However, many people find it convenient to exercise on the fast days for the first 10 days."

Varady conducted a 12-week analysis of intermittent fasting paired with endurance exercise (brisk walking/cycling) in one of the first trials to incorporate fasting and exercise interventions. Obese study participants who fasted on alternating days came to the lab three times a week to work out on stationary bikes and treadmills. When given the option of exercising on "feast" or "quick" days, participants preferred to exercise on fast days almost as much as they did on feast days.

Varady's study suggests that if weight loss is your primary target, you can wait until after work out to eat on an alternate fast day. Participants who ate their one allocated fast day meal before exercising experienced a burst of hunger an hour or so later, prompting them to cheat and eat additional calories that day.

8.27. Is it okay to have a cheat day?

It's important to be adaptable. Intermittent fasting should be seen as a way of life rather than a fad diet. , people should not be concerned if they skip 2 or 3 fast days in a month. It could be more frustrating to strictly adhere to the fast than to eat a piece of cake if your fast days fall on a holiday or during a family event.

On the other hand, some people think that "cheating" throws their whole fasting routine off. Varady recommends not skipping the fast days for family gatherings or other occasions if you are the sort of person who requires a lot of preparation to excel at a healthy activity. However, most people won't notice a big difference in their weight loss or metabolic health if they have a cheat day now and then.

8.28. Does intermittent fasting promote longevity?

Animal studies have shown that dietary restriction, such as caloric restriction and intermittent fasting, can extend healthy lifespan and delay disease aging in various species ranging from yeast to mice to monkeys. The removal or functional improvement of senescent cells, or weakened cells that have been identified by the body and stopped from dividing, is one of the biological mechanisms of these effects. Intermittent fasting can prepare senescent cells for recycling, which could help aging tissues function better.

However, studying aging and senescence cell in humans is difficult, particularly since most people are unable or unwilling to engage in long-term intervention studies. Human data from such experiments are uncommon, and the areas of caloric restriction and intermittent fasting are no exception.

Intermittent fasting (IF) can better tissue function, especially in circadian rhythms and metabolic function. Further research on the effects of long-term fasting on lifespan and healthspan is required.

8.29. How long is it safe to fast?

Clinical studies show that water fasts of up to 24-36 hours are usually healthy and well-tolerated. However, 24-hr water fasting daily for weight - loss can be difficult to implement as a lengthy health practice. Without the supervision of a physician, women with eating disorders also shouldn't practice IF. On the other hand, alternate-day fasting has been shown to reduce stress and binge eating behavior in obese people while enhancing body image perceptions.

If you feel light-headedness or extreme pain, or if you're at risk of being underweight, you should avoid fasting and see a doctor. Intermittent fasting isn't the only way to boost your metabolic health; you can also figure out what kind of meals and when they should be eaten. There is no research on the long-term effects or safety of fasting for 3 to 5 days at a time.

8.30. Can fasting impact bone density?

There's no evidence that fasting is bad for your bones. In a postmenopausal women's research, DEXA scans revealed that six months of fasting did not affect bone density.

Should I be concerned about the effects of missing meals on my blood glucose levels?

Breakfast missing (front-end fasting) has been linked to an acute state of muscular glucose resistance when refeeding. Based on normal daily cycles of insulin sensitivity, there is some evidence that missing dinner or beginning an extended overnight fast early in the evening is preferable to skipping breakfast or fast until late in the afternoon. Acute fasting studies that look at the effects of 24- to 48-hour fasts on people who aren't used to fasting for this long aren't always representative of what happens to people (who fast regularly). Based on cellular modifications to fasting stress, study participants undergo significant reductions in sugar levels and insulin resistance after a month of alternate-day fasting.

8.31. Will I lose muscle if I practice intermittent fasting long-term?

Intermittent fasting can result in lean mass and fat loss over time. However, some evidence shows that losing weight via IF may result in less muscle loss than conventional dieting or caloric restriction compared to fat loss. Intermittent fasting may result in an equal or smaller amount of muscle loss, or 10%, compared to conventional dieting without exercise, resulting in 75 percent fat loss and 25% muscle loss. When you lose weight, though, you will still lose some muscle mass. Regular physical activity, especially resistance training or weight-bearing, can prevent muscle loss during IF diets.

8.32. Who can most benefit from intermittent fasting?

Intermittent fasting study for diabetes (type 2) or at risk for diabetes (type 2) is only in its early stages, with most of the work being done in animal models. However, Dr. Krista Varady's lab has produced promising pilot study results linked to increased glucose control over time. According to recent research, intermittent fasting (IF) has a greater beneficial effect on insulin resistance than conventional calorie restriction diets. Pre-diabetics and diabetics may benefit the most from IF, but further research is required.

Both pre-diabetics and diabetics should consult with their healthcare provider before and during any form of fasting, as it may affect their drug needs and other symptoms.

Additional Intermittent Fasting Suggestions

Aim for 12-16 hours of calorie-free time.

To allow your body to burn fat between meals, avoid snacking between meals and at night.

Maintain a high level of activity during the day to aid muscle development.

During fasting periods, drink water or a calorie-free beverage to remain hydrated and relieve cravings and hunger.

You can drink coffee or tea during your fasting time if they are part of your daily routine.

Don't binge after fasting; instead, feed until you're satisfied, but not too much.

Wait out the hunger pangs; they'll pass.

Chapter No 9: Recommended Foods and Recipes For Intermittent Fasting

9.1 Best Foods to Eat While Intermittent Fasting

Intermittent fasting has gotten a lot of attention recently as one of the most popular fad diets. Fasting has been used as a form of dissent, a desire for spiritual reward, and a therapeutic tool throughout history. It's also recently gained popularity among fitness gurus due to its claimed weight-loss and anti-aging effects. But this leads to the question: Is there a detailed intermittent fasting guide that will inform you what to eat and when to eat it?

Let's start from the beginning and go over the fundamentals: In terms of these big intermittent fasting health benefits, how does the diet work? Scientists agree that improved insulin sensitivity is responsible for the anti-aging effects, although weight loss is linked to a lower average calorie intake due to a shorter feeding window. Simply put, you eat less because you have less time to eat during the day. Isn't that easy? But, as with any diet, deciding if it is feasible for your lifestyle is important.

Diet-induced weight loss usually results in a 70 percent weight gain, according to a report published in The Lancet Diabetes & Endocrinology, so finding a weight-loss strategy that works for you and won't harm you in the future is crucial.

The time-restricted feeding (TRF) solution, according to Andres Ayesta, RDN, MS, specialist and registered dietitian in the fasting field, is the best choice for working adults.

"Fasting from 9 p.m. to around 1 p.m. the next day does well because most people miss breakfast or eat bad breakfast," Ayesta notes. This method can be used around a day job, but Ayesta stresses the importance of fulfilling dietary requirements during this time-limited feeding window. It means that while intermittent fasting, overall diet consistency and habitual food preferences still matter, and you're unlikely to achieve your ideal body by eating only hamburgers and fries. In reality, on the IF diet, eating junk food during a condensed feeding window can put you at risk of deficiency in key nutrients like calcium, iron, protein, and fiber, all necessary for normal biological function. Furthermore, a diet rich in fruits and vegetables helps your body produce more antioxidants, which, like the metabolic benefits of intermittent fasting, can help you live longer.

Here's a review of typical intermittent fasting plans to get you started:

- Alternate Day Fasting (ADF) consists of one day of ad libitum (normal eating) followed by one day of full fasting.

- 1 day of ad libitum eating alternated with 1 day of an extremely low-calorie diet is known as modified alternate-day fasting (mADF) (about 25 % of normal caloric intake)

- 2/5—2 days of complete fasting followed by 5 days of ad libitum feeding

- 1/6—1 day of full fasting followed by 6 days of ad libitum feeding

Time Restricting Feeding (TRF) entails fasting for 12-20 hours a day on each day of the week (as a continuation of the nighttime fast). "Feeding window" of 4-12 hours Okay, so you know when you should eat, but you probably think about what to eat during the IF journey. A list of 20 of the healthiest meals for an intermittent fasting diet guide will help you avoid nutrient deficiency.

1. Water

Promoting hydration is one of the most critical aspects of maintaining a balanced eating routine during intermittent fasting. After going without food for 12 to 16 hours, the body's preferred energy source is the sugar contained in the liver, also defined as glycogen. As this energy is consumed, a significant amount of fluid and electrolytes is wasted. During the intermittent fasting regimen, drink at least 8 cups of water a day to stop dehydration and boost cognition, blood flow, and muscle and joint support.

2. Coffee

How about a hot cup of tea? Will a regular trip to Starbucks be enough to break the fast? It's a concern that many newbie intermittent fasters have. But don't worry: coffee is allowed. Coffee should legally be drunk outside of a given feeding window because it is a calorie-free drink in its natural state. However, once creamers, syrups, or candied flavors are added, the drink can no longer be taken during the fast, so keep that in mind if you like to doctor up your drink.

3. Minimally-Processed Grains

Carbohydrates are a necessary part of life and are not the problem when it comes to losing weight. Since you'll be fasting for a large portion of the day during this diet, it is important to plan ahead of time to get enough calories without feeling bloated. While a balanced diet avoids refined foods, there is a place and time for bagels, whole-grain bread, and crackers, which digest more easily and provide quick and easy energy. These will be a perfect source of energy on the go if you intend to work out or train regularly during intermittent fasting.

4. Raspberries

The 2015-2020 Dietary Guidelines called fiber (a shortfall nutrient)—the stuff that keeps you regular, and a recent piece of writing in Nutrients reported that less than 10% of Western populations eat sufficient amounts of whole fruits. Raspberry is a tasty, high-fiber fruit that will keep you regular during the shortened feeding window, with eight grams of fiber per cup.

5. Lentils

With 32 %of total daily fiber needs met in just half a cup, this healthy superstar is a fiber powerhouse. Lentils are a good source of iron (about 15% of your daily needs), which is another nutrient of interest, especially for active females who fast.

6. Potatoes

White potatoes, like bread, digest quickly with little effort on the part of the body. They're also a great post-workout snack when combined with a protein source to refresh hungry muscles. Another advantage of potatoes for the IF diet is that they form a resistant starch that fuels healthy bacteria in your gut when they are cooled.

7. Seitan

For optimum health and longevity, the EAT-Lancet Commission recently published a study calling for a significant reduction of animal-based proteins. One major study found a direct correlation between red meat consumption and increased mortality. Incorporate life-extending plant-based protein replacements like seitan into your anti-aging diet. This food, also described as "wheat meat," can be baked, battered, and dipped in various sauces.

8. Hummus

Hummus, one of the tastiest and creamiest dips ever made, is another outstanding plant-based protein that can be used to improve the nutritional quality of everyday foods like sandwiches by simply substituting it for mayonnaise. If you're able to make hummus, don't forget that garlic and tahini are the main ingredients.

9. Salmon Caught in the Wild

Dietary and lifestyle choices linked to extreme longevity are well established in these 5 geographical regions in Asia, Latin America, Europe, and the United States. Salmon, which is high in the brain-boosting omega-3 fatty acids EPA and DHA, is common throughout these areas.

10. Soybeans

Isoflavones, one of the active compounds in soybeans, have been shown to prevent UVB-induced cell damage and promote anti-aging. So, the next time you have a dinner party at home, impress the guests with a tasty soybean recipe.

11. Multivitamins

One of the mechanisms for why IF causes weight loss is that the person has less food to eat and therefore consumes less calories. Although the concept of energy in versus energy out holds, the possibility of vitamin deficiencies while in a caloric deficit is rarely discussed. Although a multivitamin isn't needed if you eat a well-balanced diet rich in fruits and vegetables, living can get hectic, but a supplement can fill in the gaps.

12. Smoothies

If a daily supplement doesn't sound appealing, consider making homemade smoothies with fruits and vegetables for a double dose of vitamins. Smoothies are an excellent way to consume a variety of foods, each of which is rich in various essential nutrients.

Easy tip: Buying frozen will save you money while still ensuring maximum freshness.

13. Milk fortified with vitamin D

A daily calcium intake of 1,000 milligrams is recommended for adults, roughly equivalent to three milk cups. With a smaller feeding window, opportunities to drink this much can be restricted, so high-calcium foods should be prioritized. Vitamin D fortified milk improves calcium absorption and helps to maintain bone strength. You can add the milk to smoothies or cereals, or simply drink it with meals, to increase the daily calcium intake. Non-dairy calcium sources include tofu and soy products, as well as leafy greens like kale if you're not a fan of the beverage.

14. Red Wine

The polyphenol in grapes has distinct anti-aging effects, so a glass of wine and a night of beauty sleep can keep heads turning. SIRT-1 is an enzyme class found in humans thought to function on resveratrol in the presence of a caloric deficit to improve insulin sensitivity and longevity.

15. Blueberries

Don't be fooled by their tiny size: Blueberries are a perfect example of how good things can come in small packets. Anti-oxidative mechanisms have been shown in research to lead to survival and youthfulness. Antioxidants are abundant in blueberries, and wild blueberries are among the highest antioxidant sources. Antioxidants aid in the removal of free radicals from the body and the protection of cellular damage.

16. Papaya

You'll probably start to feel hungry in the final hrs of the fast, particularly if you're new to intermittent fasting. This "hanger" can lead to you overeating in large amounts, leaving you bloated and tired minutes later. Papain, a special enzyme found in papaya, works on proteins to grind them down. Incorporating chunks of this sweet fruit into a high-protein meal will aid digestion and avoid bloating.

17. Nuts

Nut intake was also linked to a lower risk of Type 2 diabetes, cardiovascular disease, and overall mortality in a prospective trial published in the British Journal of Nutrition.

18. Ghee

You don't want to cook with an oil that has reached its smoke point, so the next time you're making a stir-fry, go with ghee. It's essentially clarified butter with a much higher smoke point, making it ideal for hot dishes.

19. Salad Dressings Made at Home

When it comes to salad dressings and sauces, you can follow your grandmother's guide and keep things plain. Extra sugar and unwanted additives are removed when we make our basic dressings.

20. Branch Chain Amino Acid Supplement

The BCAA is a final IF-approved supplement. Although this muscle-building supplement is best for those who enjoy fasted cardio or intense workouts first thing in the morning, it can also be consumed during the day (fasting or not) to keep the body from being catabolic, maintaining lean muscle mass. Note that this supplement might be off-limits if you adopt a vegan diet since it is made from duck feathers.

9.2 Breakfast Recipes

1. Spinach Parmesan Baked Eggs Recipe

Cook Time: 20 mins Prep Time: 10 mins Servings: 1

Ingredients

- 2 tsp olive oil
- 1 tomato small, diced small
- 2 garlic cloves minced
- 4 eggs
- 4 cups baby spinach
- 1/2 cup fat-free parmesan cheese, grated

Instructions

1. Preheat the oven to 350 degrees Fahrenheit. Using a nonstick spray, coat an 8-inch by 8-inch casserole dish.

2. Heat the oil in a big skillet over medium heat. Toss the garlic and spinach once the pan is warmed. Cook until the spinach is fully wilted. Remove the pan from the heat and drain any remaining liquid. Stir in the parmesan cheese, then spoon the mixture into the casserole dish in an even layer.

3. For the eggs, make four tiny divots in the spinach. Crack 1 egg into every divot. Bake for 15 to 20 minutes, or until the egg whites are almost fully set. Remove from the oven and set aside to cool for 5 minutes before adding the tomato. Serve and have fun!

2. Hummus Breakfast Bowl

Cook Time: 10 mins Prep Time: 10 mins Servings: 1

Ingredients

- 2 tbsp bell pepper any color, minced
- 1 tsp sunflower seeds
- 1 cup kale stems removed, leaves roughly chopped
- 2 egg whites
- 1/4 cup Roma tomatoes diced small
- 1 tbsp hummus
- 1 tbsp olive oil
- 1/4 cup brown rice or quinoa, cooked

Instructions

1. Heat the oil in a big skillet on medium heat. When the pan is warmed, add the kale.
2. After 3-4 minutes, add the peppers and tomatoes to the kale. Add another 4-5 minutes to the cooking time.
3. Lightly whisk the egg before gradually adding the peppers and kale. Scramble the eggs until they're no longer runny.
4. Fill a serving bowl halfway with quinoa or rice, then top with an egg and vegetables. Sprinkle the sunflower seeds on top of the hummus. Have fun!

3. Protein Pancakes

Cook Time: 10 mins Prep Time: 15 mins Servings: 1

Ingredients

- 1/4 tsp baking powder
- 1/2 cup banana mashed
- 3 egg whites
- 1 tbsp vanilla protein powder optional, chocolate protein powder

Instructions

1. Whisk together all of the ingredients in a bowl until smooth.
2. Heat a skillet over medium heat, lightly sprayed with nonstick spray. 1/4 cup batter should be poured into the tub. Cook for almost 3 to 4 minutes, or until the middle of the pancakes begins to bubble. Cook again for almost 2 to 3 minutes after carefully flipping. Remove the pancake from the pan until it is fully cooked and repeat it until all batters are used. In between pancakes, spray the skillet with nonstick spray as needed.
3. Honey, fresh fruit or the favorite nut butter can be added to the top! Have fun!

4. Egg and Ham Breakfast Cups

Cook Time: 10 mins Prep Time: 20 mins Servings: 1

Ingredients

- 2 slices low-sodium ham, all-natural

- 1/4 cup skim milk
- 1 green onions chopped
- 1 egg
- 1 egg whites

Instructions

1. Preheat the oven to 350 degrees Fahrenheit.

2. Using a nonstick spray, lightly coat a muffin tin. Each ham slice should be pressed into a cup shape in the muffin pan.

3. Whisk together the egg whites, egg, and milk in a mixing bowl. Add the green onion and fill the ham cups to about 3/4 capacity.

4. Bake for about 20 minutes or until the eggs are fully set. Remove from the oven and set aside to cool a little before serving. Have fun!

5. No-Bake Oatmeal Raisin Energy Bites

Cook Time: 10 mins Prep Time: 30 mins Servings: 12 Energy bites

Ingredients

- 1 tbsp vanilla protein powder
- 1/4 cup peanut butter
- 1/2 tsp ground cinnamon
- 2 tbsp honey
- 1/4 cup peanuts chopped
- 1/4 cup semisweet mini chocolate chips
- 1 cup dry oats
- 1/4 cup raisins

Instructions

1. Combine all ingredients in a large mixing bowl and stir until well mixed and sticky.

2. Roll into 1" balls and put on a baking sheet lined with parchment paper. Refrigerate for approximately 30 minutes or until solid. Store in an airtight jar, covered and refrigerated.

6. Creamy Green Smoothie with a Hint of Mint

Cook Time: 0 mins Prep Time: 5 mins Servings: 1

Ingredients

- 4 to 6 ice wedges
- 5 cubes of honeydew melon, 1" cubes
- 2 mint leaves fresh, more for garnish
- 1/2 avocado seeded, ripe and peeling removed
- 1/2 cups buttermilk low fat

- 1 frozen banana ripe, sliced before freezing
- 3 romaine heart leaves
- 2 tsp honey optional

Instructions

1. In a blender, combine all ingredients and blend until creamy and smooth. If needed, add 2 tsp whipped topping. For a delicious addition, try the 100 percent Clean Whipped Topping!
2. If needed, top with cinnamon and serve.

7. Sweet Potato Breakfast Hash

Cook Time: 15 mins Prep Time: 10 mins Servings: 1

Ingredients

- 1 tsp honey
- 2 sweet potatoes large, peeled and diced small
- 1 avocado peeled, pit removed and diced small
- 3 tbsp olive oil
- 1 tbsp lemon juice
- 1/2 tsp kosher salt
- 2 ounces ham low-sodium, sulfate-free, diced small
- 1/4 tsp ground white pepper
- 1/4 cup green bell pepper diced small
- 2 garlic cloves minced
- 1 tbsp apple cider vinegar
- 1/4 cup yellow onion diced small

Instructions

1. Preheat the oven to 450 degrees Fahrenheit. Using foil, line a baking sheet.
2. Toss 1/2 tbsp olive oil, the diced sweet potatoes, pepper, and salt spread out on the baking sheet in an even layer. Bake for 15 minutes, or until the potatoes are soft and lightly browned.
3. In a small cup, combine the apple cider vinegar, garlic, and honey. Add 1 tbsp extra-virgin olive oil while whisked continuously. Mix until it's combined well. Set aside.
4. Heat the remaining olive oil in a large skillet over medium heat. Add the green pepper and onion once the pan is heated. Cook until the onions start to soften, and add cooked potatoes and ham. Continue cooking until the ham starts to brown. Take the pan off the heat and add the apple cider vinegar sauce.
5. Combine the lemon juice and avocado in a mixing bowl. Stir gently into the hash. Serve warm!

9.3 Lunch Recipes

1. Oven-Crisp Fish Tacos

Cook Time: 13 mins Prep Time: 10 mins Servings: 1

Ingredients

- 1/2 pounds fish filets
- 1/4 cup whole-wheat bread crumbs
- 2 tbsp freshly squeezed lime juice, 1 medium lime
- 1/2 cup yogurt nonfat (Greek), optional nonfat sour cream
- 1/4 cup whole-wheat flour (white)
- ¼ cup cabbage or lettuce shredded
- 1 egg white
- 1 cup salsa (no sugar added) or 1 medium tomato, diced
- wide strips (3 or 4 strips per fillet)
- 2 corn tortillas 6 inches or whole- wheat flour tortillas
- 1/4 cup cornmeal
- 2 tbsp taco seasoning recipe for homemade Taco Seasoning

Instructions

1. Preheat the oven to 450 degrees Fahrenheit.
2. By using a foil, cover a baking sheet. Spray a rack with canola oil or olive oil spray and place it on top of the baking sheet.
3. In a small cup, combine cornmeal, taco seasoning, and breadcrumbs.
4. Mix the lime juice and egg whites in a separate shallow bowl until frothy.
5. Put flour in a deep bowl.
6. To finely coat both sides of the fish strips, gently dip them into the flour. Dip the fish pieces in the egg whites, allowing excess to fall away, then press the fish pieces on both sides into the breadcrumbs and seasoned cornmeal.
7. Cook the breaded fish pieces for almost 10 to 12 minutes on the prepared rack until the outside is crispy and the fish is smooth and breaks easily with a fork.
8. Coat a griddle or a saute pan with cooking oil. Heat the tortillas on both sides over medium heat for 30 secs to 1 minute, or until thoroughly cooked. Until ready to eat, keep tortillas hot in a clean kitchen towel.
9. Place 2 pieces of the fish into every tortilla, top with salsa or tomato, shredded romaine, and yogurt.

2. Asparagus Foil Pack and Baked Lemon Salmon

Cook Time: 15 mins Prep Time: 10 mins Servings: 4

Ingredients

- 16 to 24 ounces salmon filets 4 pieces
- 2 tbsp lemon zest
- 1 pound asparagus fresh, about 1 inch of the bottom ends trimmed off
- 2 tbsp parsley fresh, chopped
- 1 tsp kosher salt
- 1 tbsp thyme fresh, chopped
- 1/2 tsp ground black pepper
- 2 tbsp olive oil
- 1/4 cup lemon juice fresh

Instructions

1. Preheat oven to 400 degrees Fahrenheit.

2. Spray 4 wide sheets of foil with nonstick spray and place on a flat surface. Place the asparagus in a single sheet, side by side, in each of the packets. Season with half of the pepper and salt.

3. On top of each asparagus bed, place a salmon fillet. Drizzle with the rest of the pepper and salt, as well as the lemon juice, olive oil, and thyme. Fold each side of the foil sheets up carefully to form a packet around the salmon and put in a layer on a baking sheet. Cook for 15 minutes in the oven

4. Remove the packets from the oven, gently open everyone, and be careful of the steam that will be emitted! On top, sprinkle parsley and lemon zest. Serve and have fun!

3. Wild Cod with Moroccan Couscous

Cook Time: 25 mins Prep Time: 5 mins Servings: 4

Ingredients

- 1/2 cup chicken broth fat-free, low sodium
- 14 1/2 ounces diced tomatoes with green chilies can
- 16 ounces wild-caught cod fillets thawed (4 fillets)
- 1 tbsp plus 2 tsp olive oil (extra virgin)
- black pepper to taste
- 3/4 cup couscous (Moroccan), whole-wheat couscous (optional)
- 1 tbsp lemon juice freshly squeezed
- sea or kosher salt to taste

Instructions

1. Add 2 tsp extra-virgin olive oil, chicken broth, and tomatoes (diced) with juice to a medium pot. Bring to a boil over medium heat, then add the couscous and season with pepper and salt. Remove from heat, then stir, and cover the saucepan. Allow the couscous to sit while you prepare the cod.

2. Season the cod with a pinch of salt and a grind of black pepper. In a big nonstick skillet, heat 1 tbsp oil over medium heat and cook the fillets until they flake with a fork, around 2-3 minutes on each side. Take the pan off the heat, then serve with couscous. Pour lemon juice over the fillets.

4. Turkey Skillet and Sweet Potato

Cook Time: 25 mins Prep Time: 5 mins Servings: 6

Ingredients

- 1 tbsp extra virgin olive oil
- 1/2 cup part-skim mozzarella cheese, grated
- 1/4 tsp pepper
- 1 pound ground turkey, leaned
- 1 medium onion, minced
- 1/2 tsp kosher or sea salt
- 2 medium sweet potatoes, diced into tiny cubes
- 1 tsp cumin
- 2 sage leaves fresh, roughly chopped

Instructions

1. Sauté the onion in a wide saucepan with olive oil over medium-low heat until soft, around 4 minutes. Cook until the turkey is no longer pink, breaking it up with a fork. Remove any excess fat. Combine the cumin, sweet potatoes, salt, sage, and pepper in a large mixing bowl. Cook, occasionally stirring, until potatoes are soft but not falling apart, around 5 to 10 minutes.

2. Drizzle the mozzarella on top of the sweet potatoes when they're tender, cover, and turn off the oven.

3. Before eating, wait until the cheese has melted.

5. Cucumber Quinoa Salad with Olives, Ground Turkey, & Feta

Cook Time: 0 mins Prep Time: 10 mins Servings: 12

Ingredients

- 1 tbsp lemon juice
- 3 cucumbers large, sliced into 1/4 inch half circles
- 1 tbsp oregano fresh, chopped
- 1 red onion small, sliced thin
- 2 garlic cloves minced
- 1 cup grape tomatoes sliced in half
- 2 tbsp mint fresh, chopped
- 1/2 cup kalamata olives
- 1/2 cup feta cheese crumbles fat-free

- 1/2 pound ground turkey sausage
- 1 1/2 cup quinoa cooked

Instructions

1. Heat the turkey sausage in a big skillet. As the sausage cooks, break it up into tiny pieces. Drain any remaining liquid and allow it to cool completely.

2. Combine the turkey sausage with the rest of the ingredients until it has cooled. Until serving, thoroughly combine all ingredients and relax. Have fun!

6. Baked Chicken and Vegetable Spring Rolls

Cook Time: 40 mins Prep Time: 20 mins Servings: 8

Ingredients

- 1 cup string beans or flat beans, ends taken away and sliced diagonally
- 3 tbsp extra virgin olive oil divided
- 8 spring roll wrappers
- 1 garlic clove finely chopped
- 1/4 tsp ground pepper
- 1 onion small, finely chopped
- 1/4 tsp salt
- 4 ounces boneless and skinless chicken breasts diced small
- 3 tbsp soy sauce low salt
- 1 cup carrots julienned
- 1 cup cabbage julienned

Instructions

1. Preheat the oven to 400 degrees Fahrenheit.

2. Sauté the onion and garlic in a wide saucepan with 2 tbsp extra virgin olive oil over medium heat for 1 minute.

3. Cook for around 5 minutes after adding the chicken.

4. Toss in all of the vegetables and cook for around 15 minutes.

5. Add the salt, soy sauce, and pepper, then toss for 1 minute. Set aside.

6. Layout 2 filo squares (1 square will instantly break) or 1 spring roll wrapper on the work surface to make the rolls. Place a portion of sautéed vegetables and chicken nearest to you. Roll, tuck in the sides and continue rolling until you reach the end. Wet your fingers with water and gently dab the filo ends to seal them. Continue to work on the remaining spring rolls.

7. Put the spring rolls on a tray covered with parchment paper.

8. Brush the remainder 1 tbsp extra-virgin olive oil over each spring roll.

9. Preheat the oven to 350 degrees F and bake for almost 15 to 20 minutes, or until lightly browned.

10. Serve with a sour and sweet sauce or some other dipping sauce of your choice.

7. Spicy Black Bean & Shrimp Salad Recipe

Cook Time: 20 mins Prep Time: 5 mins Servings: 2

Ingredients

- 1 tsp chili powder
- 2 cups kale shredded or finely chopped
- 1/2 tsp kosher salt
- 1 avocado peeled and pit removed and sliced
- 1 tbsp lime juice
- 1 tsp smoked paprika
- 1 tsp ground cumin
- 1/4 cup red onion diced small
- 2 tbsp cilantro fresh, chopped
- 1 cup corn kernels
- 2 cup romaine lettuce shredded or finely chopped
- 1/2 pound shrimp large, raw, peeled and deveined
- 15 ounces black beans drained and rinsed
- 2 tbsp olive oil
- 1/4 tsp crushed red pepper
- 1 cup grape tomatoes cut in half

Instructions

1. Combine the red pepper, shrimp, chili powder, cumin, paprika, and salt in a small cup. Toss the shrimp in the seasonings thoroughly.

2. In a big skillet, heat 1 tbsp of olive oil. Put the seasoned shrimp once the pan is hot. Cook for almost 5 to 6 minutes, or until the meat is firm and pink. Keep the shrimp warm after removing them from the skillet.

3. Return the shrimp to the pan with the left tbsp of olive oil. Heat on high and add the onion and corn once the pan is warmed. Cook until the corn starts to char and the onions are tender, for around 5 minutes. Combine the black beans, lime juice, and cooked shrimp in a mixing bowl. Cook for just a few minutes or until the beans are sweet.

4. Toss the romaine and kale together in a big salad bowl. Add the tomato, shrimp mixture, and avocado to the top. Serve with a sprinkling of cilantro on top.

9.4 Dinner Recipes

1. Easy Turkey Burrito Skillet

Cook Time: 15 mins Prep Time: 5 mins Servings: 6

Ingredients

- 1/4 cup water
- 1 pound ground turkey
- 1/4 cup cilantro fresh, chopped
- 1 tbsp chili powder
- 1/2 cup Greek yogurt plain
- 1 tsp ground cumin
- 1 cup low-fat cheddar cheese
- 1 tbsp lime juice
- 4 whole-wheat flour tortillas 6 inches, cut into 1-inch strips
- 1/2 tsp kosher salt
- 15 ounces of black beans can (drained and rinsed)
- 1/4 tsp ground black pepper (or crushed red pepper if you like it spicy!)
- 1 cup chunky salsa no sugar added

Instructions

1. Cook the ground turkey in a large skillet until it is cooked through, breaking it up into small pieces as it heats. Cumin, chili powder, salt, lime juice, pepper, salsa, water, and beans should all be mixed. Bring to a boil, then lower to low heat. Cook, occasionally stirring, for 3 to 5 minutes, or until the sauce thickens.

2. Remove the pan from the heat and add the tortilla strips, followed by the shredded cheese. Cover and keep warm until the cheese has melted. Serve with a dollop of Greek yogurt and a sprig of fresh cilantro on top of each serving. Serve and have fun!

2. Chicken and Broccoli Stir-Fry

Cook Time: 25 mins Prep Time: 5 mins Servings: 4

Ingredients

- 2 cups broccoli florets
- 1 tbsp extra virgin olive oil
- 1/4 tsp black pepper
- 1 onion medium, coarsely chopped
- 2 tsp sesame seeds
- 3 tbsp lite soy sauce optional tamari
- 1 1-inch ginger root finely chopped and peeled
- 1 tbsp honey
- 2 tsp lemon juice
- 2 tbsp sesame oil

- 1 tbsp cornstarch or flour
- 1 1/4 pounds skinless and boneless chicken breasts cubed

Instructions

1. Combine the honey, soy sauce, sesame oil, lemon juice, and cornstarch in a mixing bowl. Set aside the mixture.

2. Toast sesame seeds in a large skillet or wok over medium-low heat for 2 minutes or until fragrant. Put aside the toasted seeds in a cup.

3. In the same skillet, heat the olive oil over medium heat and cook the chicken until it is lightly golden. Combine the onions, broccoli, ginger, and pepper in a large mixing bowl. Reduce the heat to medium-low and toss in the soy sauce mixture. Cook for almost 5 minutes, or until sauce reaches target thickness. Serve with toasted sesame seeds. Have fun!

4. Enjoy chicken & broccoli stir-fry with quinoa or brown rice in a skillet.

3. Honey Garlic Shrimp Stir-Fry

Cook Time: 10 mins Prep Time: 10 mins Servings: 4

Ingredients

- 1 tbsp coconut oil
- 2 cups brown rice cooked
- 1 pound shrimp peeled, raw and deveined
- 1 tbsp orange zest
- 2 garlic cloves minced
- 1 tbsp soy sauce
- 1 tbsp fresh ginger, minced
- 2 tbsp honey
- 1 small yellow onion, cut into thin strips
- 1/2 tsp kosher salt
- 1 small red bell pepper, cut into thin strips
- 1 cup peas

Instructions

1. Heat the coconut oil in a large skillet over high heat. Add half of the garlic, the shrimp, and half of the ginger once the pan is heated. Cook until the shrimp are solid, stirring constantly. Remove the shrimp from the pan and set them aside.

2. Add the onion, bell pepper, snap peas, and the remaining ginger and garlic to the same pan where the shrimp was cooked. Cook on high heat, stirring continuously until the vegetables begin to soften.

3. Return the shrimp to the pan, add soy sauce, honey, orange zest, and salt season. Cook until all of the ingredients are hot and well-coated in the sauce. Serve with brown rice and eat up!

4. Savory Lemon Fish Fillets

Cook Time: 15 mins Prep Time: 15 mins Servings: 4

Ingredients

- 1/4 tsp sea or kosher salt
- 2 lemons, one cut in wedges, one cut in halves
- 3 tbsp olive oil
- 16 to 22 ounces cod fillets halibut
- 1/4 tsp freshly ground black pepper

Instructions

1. Allow the fish to rest for 10 to 15 minutes in a bowl at room temperature.

2. On both sides of each fillet, rub 1 tbsp olive oil and season with salt and pepper. Add two tbsp of olive oil to a sauté pan or a skillet over medium heat. After about one minute, when the oil is hot and shimmering but not smoking, add the fish. Cook for 2 to 3 minutes on both sides, until the fish, is golden brown and cooked through.

3. Remove the fish from the heat after squeezing both lemon halves over it. If there is any remaining lemon juice in the pan, drizzle it over the fish before serving. Serve with lemon wedges on the side.

5. Skinny Salmon, Kale, & Cashew Bowl

Cook Time: 15 mins Prep Time: 10 mins Servings: 6

Ingredients

- 1/4 tsp kosher salt
- 2 tbsp olive oil
- 1/2 tsp lemon zest
- 1/2 tsp kosher salt
- 1 garlic clove finely grated or minced
- 1/4 tsp ground black pepper
- 1 tsp lemon juice
- 2 minced garlic cloves
- 3/4 cup Greek yogurt
- 4 cups kale stems removed and chopped
- Optional Lemon Yogurt Sauce
- 1/2 cup carrots shredded
- 1/4 cup cashews chopped
- 2 cups quinoa cooked (according to package)
- 12 ounces salmon skinless

Instructions

1. Preheat the oven to 400 degrees Fahrenheit and prepare a baking sheet with parchment paper. Spread the salmon fillets out on the baking sheet. Season the salmon with salt and pepper after brushing it with 1 tbsp of oil (reserve the other tbsp for later). Preheat the oven to 350 degrees F and bake for 15 minutes, or until firm and flaky.

2. Meanwhile, in a pan, heat the remaining oil. Add the kale, garlic, and carrot once the pan is warmed. Cook until the kale is wilted and gentle, stirring frequently. Combine the cashews and quinoa in a mixing bowl. Cook, constantly stirring until the mixture is hot.

3. Fill a serving bowl halfway with the quinoa and kale mixture. Place the salmon on top of the kale after it has been removed from the oven. Serve and have fun.

9.5 Snacks and Appetizers Recipes

1. Skinny Turkey Meatloaf

Cook Time: 45 mins Prep Time: 5 mins Servings: 8

Ingredients

- 1 lb lean ground turkey recommend 93% lean
- 1/3 cup ketchup
- 1 egg lightly whipped with a fork
- 1/4 tsp salt
- 1/3 cup rolled oats uncooked
- 1/2 tsp black pepper
- 1/3 cup chunky salsa no sugar added
- 1/2 cup onion diced

Instructions

1. Preheat the oven to 375 degrees Fahrenheit.

2. In a mixing bowl, combine all ingredients except the ketchup. Fill a 5 x 7-inch loaf pan halfway with the mixture and press to make a loaf. Bake for 35 minutes.

3. Remove the pan from the oven and uniformly spread the ketchup on top. Bake for another 10 minutes.

4. Allow for a 5-minute rest period. Remove the whole loaf from the pan, put it on a serving platter, and slice the loaf first.

2. Easy Turkey Sausage with Peppers & Onions

Cook Time: 15 mins Prep Time: 10 mins Servings: 4

Ingredients

- 1 cup sliced green pepper
- 1 pound turkey rope sausage, sliced into thick half-moons
- 1 cup sliced red onion
- 1/2 tbsp olive oil
- 1 cup sliced yellow pepper

Instructions

1. Combine all of the ingredients in a large skillet over medium-high heat. Cook, often stirring until the peppers and onions soften.

2. Serve with brown rice or quinoa as a side dish. Have fun!

3. Easy Veggie Mini Quiches

Cook Time: 25 mins Prep Time: 10 mins Servings: 24

Ingredients

*   2 green shallots (onions), green ends trimmed off, white finely chopped (optional)
*   ¼ tsp salt
*   ¾ cup packed green zucchini (grated)
*   ⅓ cup Monterrey Jack cheese (grated)
*   ¾ cup packed grated carrots
*   2 tsp coconut oil (or any oil)
*   4 large eggs, whisked

Instructions

1. Preheat the oven to 350 degrees Fahrenheit and grease a small cupcake pan.

2. Heat the oil in a medium bowl. Cook, occasionally stirring, for 5-7 minutes, or until the carrots, zucchini, and shallots soften. Take the pan off the heat and set it aside to cool to room temperature.

3. Combine the vegetables, grated cheese, eggs, and salt in a big mixing bowl. Fill mini muffin tins halfway with the mixture.

4. Preheat the oven to 150 degrees Fahrenheit and bake for 15 to 18 minutes. Allow tiny quiches to cool in the skillet before removing them carefully with a knife or spatula.

4. Roasted Veggies and Savory Oats Bowl

Cook Time: 30 mins Prep Time: 10 mins Servings: 4

Ingredients

*   1 tsp black pepper, divided
*   16-ounce bag butternut squash, cubed
*   2 strips cooked turkey bacon, crumbled
*   8 ounces Brussels sprouts, halved
*   4 eggs
*   1 tbsp olive oil
*   ½ cup Sharp Cheddar cheese, shredded
*   1 tsp salt, divided
*   2 cups Quaker Old Fashioned Oats
*   1 tbsp butter

- ½ cup onion, chopped coarsely
- 2 cups water

Instructions

1. Preheat the oven to 400 degrees Fahrenheit. Using parchment paper, line a broad baking sheet.
2. Toss the butternut squash, Brussels sprouts, chopped onion, olive oil, 1/2 tsp black pepper, and 1/2 tsp salt together in a big mixing bowl, then move to the baking sheet.
3. Bake for almost 20 to 22 minutes, or until vegetables are golden brown and tender.
4. Melt the butter in a medium pot over medium heat while the vegetables roast. To toast the oats, add them to the pan and cook for 30 seconds. Bring the water to a low boil, then reduce to low heat. Reduce to low heat and continue to cook for 8 to 10 minutes or until the oats hit a thick consistency. Season with the remaining black pepper and salt and stir in the shredded cheese. Keep it warm.
5. Cook the eggs sunny-side up in a big greased nonstick pan.
6. Fill a bowl with oats, then top with vegetables, bacon crumbles, and an egg.

5. Spinach & Bacon Mini Quiches

Cook Time: 18 mins Prep Time: 5 mins Servings: 24

Ingredients

- 1 cup cheddar cheese, shredded
- 6 eggs
- Dash of pepper
- ¾ cup finely chopped spinach
- 3 tbsp milk
- 4 strips bacon, cooked and chopped

Instructions

1. Preheat the oven to 350 degrees Fahrenheit (180 degrees Celsius) and grease a mini muffin pan.
2. Whisk together the eggs and milk in a big mixing bowl. Combine the shredded cheddar, chopped spinach, pepper, and chopped bacon in a mixing bowl. To combine all of the ingredients, give it a quick stir.
3. Fill muffin pan cups halfway with egg mixture.
4. Bake for 15-18 minutes in a preheated oven.
5. Allow small quiches to cool in the skillet before carefully removing them with a knife or spatula once they are finished.

6. Cauliflower Shrimp Fried Rice

Cook Time: 10 mins Prep Time: 10 mins Servings: 4

Ingredients

- 1 tbsp sesame oil
- 6 cups cauliflower rice or 1 large head of cauliflower
- ½ pound shrimp, peeled, thawed and deveined
- ¼ cup Reduced Sodium Tamari, soy sauce or Coconut Aminos
- 3 eggs, beaten
- 1 tbsp honey
- ½ cup carrots, cubed
- ⅛ tsp ginger ground or ½ tsp fresh ginger grated
- ½ cup frozen peas
- red pepper flakes
- 1 bunch chopped green onions, whites removed from greens

Instructions

1. Cauliflower should be chopped into pieces and placed in a food processor. Pulse to chop until it looks like rice, set aside.

2. Set aside a small bowl containing San-J Tamari, ginger, honey, and red pepper flakes.

3. Heat sesame oil in a big skillet or wok over medium-high heat. Sauté for a minute after adding the white portion of the onions. Stir in the carrots and frozen peas, then heat up for around 2 minutes. Transfer the vegetables to 1 side of the pan and pour in the beaten eggs. Keep cooking eggs on 1 side of the pan until finished, turning the mixture around when it heats. Cook for about 2 minutes, or until the shrimp have turned pink.

4. Stir in the riced cauliflower until everything is well combined. Pour the Tamari sauce combination over the top, making sure it is uniformly distributed, and cook for another 4 minutes, or until the cauliflower has softened and is also firm. Turn off the heat, add the green onions, and cover for 1 minute to soften.

7. Mediterranean Chicken Farro Bowls

Cook Time: 35 mins Prep Time: 10 mins Servings: 4

Ingredients

For the bowls

- 3 cups water or stock
- 1 cup Bob's Red Mill Farro, cooked
- Lemon wedges, for serving
- ½ tsp salt
- ½ cup crumbled feta cheese
- 1 pound skinless, boneless chicken breasts (2 large breasts))
- 1 cup tzatziki sauce

- 3 tbsp olive oil
- ½ red onion, sliced
- Zest of 1 lemon
- 1 cup kalamata olives, pitted and sliced
- 2 tbsp lemon juice
- 2 cups chopped cucumber
- 2 cloves garlic, grated
- 1-pint cherry tomatoes halved
- 1 tsp dried oregano
- 1 tbsp olive oil
- ½ tsp kosher salt
- ¼ tsp black pepper
- Fresh dill and parsley, for garnish, optional

Tzatziki sauce

- 1 cup plain yogurt
- ½ tsp salt
- 1 cucumber
- ¼ tsp dried dill
- 1 garlic clove
- ½ tsp lemon juice

Instructions

1. Farro should be rinsed and drained. In a pot, combine the farro, salt, and enough water or stock to cover it. Bring to a boil, then reduce to medium-low heat and cook for 30 minutes. Any excess water should be drained.

2. For the chicken, prepare as follows: Combine olive oil, chicken breasts, lemon juice, lemon zest, garlic, salt, oregano, and pepper in a zip bag. Marinate for 4 hours or overnight.

3. Heat the olive oil in a large skillet over medium-high heat, then add the chicken breasts and cook for 7 minutes, flipping halfway through, until the internal temperature reaches 165 degrees. Remove the marinade and discard it.

4. Remove the chicken from the pan and set it aside to cool for 5 minutes before cutting.

5. Put a layer of farro at the bottom of the bowl or a container to assemble the Greek bowls. Top with sliced chicken, cucumber, tomatoes, red onion, olives, feta cheese and tzatziki sauce. Sprinkle dill and some parsley and serve with lemon wedges.

8. Super Greens Kale Salad with Sesame Ginger Dressing

Cook Time: 0 mins Prep Time: 5 mins Servings: 6

Ingredients

For the Salad

- 1 cup shelled edamame, thawed if using frozen
- 6 cups chopped kale (about 1 large head)
- ¼ cup sunflower seeds
- 2 cups red cabbage, shredded
- 1 cup shredded carrots
- ½ cup thinly sliced red onion

For the Sesame Ginger Dressing

- ½ cup rice vinegar
- 1 ½ tsp sesame oil
- ¼ cup soy sauce
- 1 garlic clove, grated
- 3 tbsp sesame seeds
- 1 tbsp brown sugar
- 2 tsp fresh ginger, grated

Instructions

1. To make the kale salad, combine all of the ingredients in a large mixing bowl
2. Layer kale, shredded carrots, red cabbage, red onion, shelled edamame, and sunflower seeds in a big mixing bowl. Serve with Sesame Ginger dressing drizzled on top.
3. To make the Sesame Ginger Dressing, combine all of the ingredients in a mixing bowl.
4. Whisk together the dressing ingredients in a big mixing bowl. Refrigerate for up to one week in a glass container.

9. Sweet potato curry with spinach and chickpeas

Cook time: 15 mins prep time: 15 mins servings: 6

Ingredients

- 1 tsp cinnamon
- 10 ounces fresh spinach, washed, stemmed and coarsely chopped
- ½ large sweet onions, chopped or 2 scallions, thinly sliced
- 1 cup chopped fresh cilantro for garnish
- 1 -2 tsp canola oil
- 1 can diced tomatoes
- 2 tbsp curry powder
- 1 cup water
- 1 tbsp cumin

- 2 large sweet potatoes, peeled and diced (about 2 lbs)
- 1 (14 1/2 ounce) can chickpeas, rinsed and drained

Instructions

1. You can bake the sweet potatoes in any way you like.
2. Chop, peel, and steam for almost 15 minutes in a veggie steamer.
3. Boiling or baking are also viable options.
4. Heat 1-2 tsp vegetable oil or canola over medium heat when sweet potatoes are cooking.
5. Add the onions and cook for 2-3 minutes, or until they soften.
6. Stir in the curry powder, cinnamon, and cumin to uniformly cover the onions in spices.
7. Stir in the tomatoes and their juices, as well as the chickpeas.
8. Increase the heat to a deep simmer for around a couple of minutes after adding 1/2 cup water.
9. Then, a few handfuls at a time, apply the fresh spinach, stirring to cover with the cooking liquid.
10. When all of the spinach has been added to the bowl, cover and cook for 3 minutes, or until just wilted.
11. Stir the cooked potatoes into the liquid to coat them.
12. Cook again for 3-5 minutes, or until all of the flavors are well mixed.
13. Serve immediately after transferring to a serving dish and tossing it with fresh cilantro.
14. This dish goes well with brown rice or basmati.

10. Poached eggs & avocado toasts

Cook time: 10 mins Prep time: 5 mins Servings: 4

Ingredients

- 4 slices thick bread
- 4 eggs
- 4 tsp butter (for spreading on toast)
- 2 ripe avocados
- salt & freshly ground black pepper
- 2 tsp lemon juice (or juice of 1 lime)
- 1 cup cheese (grated, edam, gruyere or whatever you have on hand)

Instructions

1. Use your preferred method to poach eggs.
2. Meanwhile, strip the stones from the avocados and cut them in half.
3. Scoop the flesh into a bowl with a spoon, then add the lemon or lime juice, salt, and pepper.
4. By using a fork, mash the potatoes roughly.
5. Toast the bread and spread it with butter.
6. Top each piece of buttered toast with the avocado mixture and a poached egg.

7. Serve immediately with a sprinkle of grated cheese with grilled or fresh tomato halves on the side.

11. Vegan fried 'fish' tacos

Cook time: 0 mins Prep time: 50 mins Servings: 8

Ingredients

- 1 tsp ground cumin
- ½ cup non-dairy milk
- 14 ounces silken tofu
- vegan mayonnaise, to serve
- 2 cups panko breadcrumbs
- 8 small tortillas
- ½ cup plain flour
- 1 ripe avocado
- ½ tsp salt
- ¼ head cabbage, finely shredded
- ½ tsp cayenne pepper
- 1 tsp smoked paprika
- vegetable oil, for frying
- Pickled onion
- 1 tbsp sugar
- 1 red onion, peeled, finely sliced
- ¼ cup apple cider vinegar
- 1 tsp salt

Instructions

1. To extract excess moisture, pat the tofu with a few pieces of kitchen paper. Split the tofu into rough 1" pieces with a knife.
2. Take a large shallow dish, combine the breadcrumbs in it.
3. In a separate large shallow cup, combine the salt, flour, cayenne, smoked paprika, and cumin.
4. In a third big shallow bowl, pour the milk.
5. Toss the tofu chunks in the flour, then the milk, then the breadcrumbs, and place them on a baking sheet.
6. Fill a shallow frying pan with vegetable oil to a depth of 1/2 inch. Place over medium heat and allow the oil to heat up – if a breadcrumb begins to bubble and brown, the oil is ready. Fry chunks of breaded tofu until golden underneath, then flip and finish cooking until golden all over. To drain, place on a baking sheet covered with kitchen paper. Repeat with the rest of the tofu.

7. For the pickled onion:

8. In a small pot, heat the apple cider vinegar, sugar, and salt until steaming. Pour the hot vinegar over the diced red onion in a bowl or jar. Allow it to soften and turn pink for at least 30 minutes.

9. Serve the warm fried tofu with pickled onion, avocado, vegan mayo, and shredded cabbage in warmed tortillas.

12. Sweet potato and black bean burrito

Cook time: 20 mins Prep time: 45 mins Servings: 8

Ingredients

- 4 garlic cloves, minced (or pressed)
- 1 tbsp minced fresh green chili pepper
- 4 tsp ground cumin
- 5 cups peeled cubed sweet potatoes
- fresh salsa
- 2 tsp other vegetable oil or 2 tsp broth
- 1 tsp salt
- 3 1/2 cups diced onions
- 2 tbsp fresh lemon juice
- 1/2 tsp salt
- 12 (10 inches) flour tortillas
- 4 tsp ground coriander
- 4 1/2 cups cooked black beans (three 15-ounce cans, drained)
- 2/3 cup lightly packed cilantro leaf

Instructions

1. Preheat the oven to 350 degrees Fahrenheit.

2. In a medium saucepan, combine the sweet potatoes, salt, and enough water to cover them.

3. Cover and move to a boil, then reduce to low heat and cook until the vegetables are tender, for around 10 minutes.

4. Drain the water and set it aside.

5. Heat the oil in a saucepan or a medium pan and add the garlic, onions, and Chile while the sweet potatoes are cooking.

6. Cover and then cook on medium-low heat, constantly mixing, for around 7 minutes, or until the onions are tender.

7. Cook, stirring regularly, for another 2 to 3 minutes after adding the cumin and coriander.

8. Take the pan off the heat, then set it aside.

9. In a food processor, mix the cilantro, black beans, salt, lemon juice, and puree and cooked sweet potatoes until smooth. Add the cooked onions and spices to the sweet potato mixture in a big mixing bowl.

10. A big baking dish should be lightly oiled.

11. Fill each tortilla with around 2/3 to 3/4 cup of the filling, roll it up, and put it seam side down in the baking dish.

12. Bake for 30 minutes, or until piping hot, covered tightly with foil.

13. Serve with salsa on top.

Bonus Chapter: 16/8 IF with Meal Plan for Women over 50

The 16:8 fasting method is a regular eating routine in which you fast for sixteen hours and eat for eight hours. This eating plan has all of the advantages of other fasting programs (plus, a recent study finds that it may decrease blood pressure). Even better, you get to choose the eating window.

So, what should be the name of that eating window? "There is truly an infinite amount of variation. It could happen at any moment. Fasting is when you don't eat for a while, "Fasting expert and author of The Complete Guide to Fasting, Jason Fung, M.D., describes.

If you can't go a day without eating something, eat it earlier in the day (8 a.m. to 4 p.m.). Eat-in the middle of the day if you want an early meal (11 a.m. to 6 p.m.). If you always go out with friends for late meals, consider shifting the eating hours later in the day (1 p.m. to 9 p.m.).

Contrary to common opinion, there are no requirements for how many meals you must fit into your day or whether or not you must have breakfast. In reality, no evidence eating breakfast makes one healthier or lose weight.

10.1 Getting Started With 16/8 Fasting

It's time to leap in—but not all in—once you've decided on a general feeding window and spoken with a specialist to ensure IF is correct for you. Vincent Pedre, a gut health specialist and functional medicine physician who recommends Intermittent Fasting to his patients, suggests beginning with a 12-hour daily fast and gradually increasing to a 16-hour fast. He says, "Reserve 20-hour and alternate-day fasts for those who have done it before."

Some experts recommend beginning with a couple of days per week and gradually increasing the fasting window from 12 to 14 to 16 hours. "It's important to pay attention to the body," Pedre adds.

Non-caloric beverages and exercise are permitted during fasting hours, even though food is prohibited. According to studies, they may also be able to prevent hunger. Black coffee, water, and unsweetened tea are liquids (skip the cream and sugar).

Furthermore, exercising while fasting will boost your body's fat-burning capabilities—but, as always, listen to your body. "If you feel very weak to exercise after fasting, take care of the diet and exercise later," Pedre suggests.

10.2 16/8 sample meal plans

Then there's the food. Yes, 16:8 fasting allows you to eat whatever you want during the feeding window, but it isn't an excuse to binge on pancakes, pizza, and Pringles.

"You should adhere to a safe, whole foods diet during your eating times," says functional-medicine expert Will Cole, D.C., IFMCP. "Since one of the advantages of fasting is that it reduces inflammation, overeating junk food during the eating window will worsen inflammation. And, given that inflammation is a factor contributing to almost all advanced health issues, it's something you'll want to keep in check."

Yes, to clean proteins, healthy fats, and whole-food carbohydrates. Miss the ultra-processed foods and the drive-thru, but don't overlook the importance of deliciousness. It's possible that spending less time on food prep and preparation would allow you to be more adventurous in the kitchen.

Depending on which eating window you select, here's an example of what to eat (when to eat it) on a 16:8 fasting diet:

Early feeding window meal plan

8 a.m.: veggie and egg scramble, side of whole-grain toast

10 a.m.: granola and yogurt

Noon: veggie and chicken stir fry

Evening: decaf tea

Midday feeding window meal plan

Morning tea or black coffee (no sugar or cream)

11 a.m.: peanut butter, banana smoothie

2 p.m.: avocado toast including pistachios

4 p.m.: almonds covered with dark chocolate

6 p.m.: turkey meatballs & tomato sauce over whole wheat pasta (or zucchini noodle)

Late feeding window meal plan

Morning tea or black coffee (no sugar or cream)

1 p.m.: pudding of blackberry chia

4 p.m.: quesadilla of black bean (bell pepper, black beans, cheese of your choice, and taco seasoning)

6 p.m.: banana

9 p.m.: vegetables, grilled salmon, and quinoa

10.3 16/8 Fasting – 14 Day Sample Meal Plan

Do you want to give the 16:8 diet a try? A 7-day meal plan with all you need to get started is included below. Lunch and dinner are served every day, with snacks in between the meals.

Week 1

Monday (Day 1)

1. Meal: Vegan chickpea salad
2. Snack: Greek yogurt
3. Meal: Cauliflower rice and Teriyaki chicken
4. Snack: Glass of wine and cheese

Tuesday (Day 2)

1. Meal: Avocado salad with chicken
2. Snack: Apricot slices with some mixed nuts
3. Meal: Pasta (Macadamia basil pesto)
4. Snack: Two chocolate chip cookies and a glass of milk

Wednesday (Day 3)

1. Meal: Tuna avocado salad
2. Snack: Apple slices with peanut butter
3. Meal: Grilled shrimp with black bean salsa and corn
4. Snack: Berries with coconut cream

Thursday (Day 4)

1. Meal: Turkey chili with cornbread
2. Snack: Almond slices and Organic edamame
3. Meal: Asian fried noodles
4. Snack: Fruit salad

Friday (Day 5)

1. Meal: Broccoli tofu salad with quinoa
2. Snack: Bowl of mixed berries and piece of dark chocolate
3. Meal: Garlic bread with hearty chicken tortilla soup
4. Snack: Banana pieces dipped in dark chocolate

Saturday (Day 6)

1. Meal: Chicken, sprouts, and quinoa Buddha bowl
2. Snack: Greek yogurt topped with raspberries
3. Meal: Tempeh quinoa salad (Mexican)
4. Snack: Watermelon pieces drizzled with sea salt

Sunday (Day 7)

1. Meal: Grilled salmon with mixed greens and brown rice
2. Snack: Pita and hummus with raw veggie sticks
3. Meal: Seared salmon with parmesan-kale salad and brown rice
4. Snack: Baked apple with cinnamon

Week 2

Monday (Day 1)

1. Meal: Broccoli tofu salad with quinoa
2. Snack: Bowl of mixed berries and piece of dark chocolate
3. Meal: Garlic bread with hearty chicken tortilla soup
4. Snack: Banana pieces dipped in dark chocolate

Tuesday (Day 2)

1. Meal: Tuna avocado salad
2. Snack: Apple slices with peanut butter
3. Meal: Grilled shrimp with black bean salsa and corn
4. Snack: Berries with coconut cream

Wednesday (Day 3)

1. Meal: Chicken, sprouts, and quinoa Buddha bowl
2. Snack: Greek yogurt topped with raspberries

3. Meal: Tempeh quinoa salad (Mexican)

4. Snack: Watermelon pieces drizzled with sea salt

Thursday (Day 4)

1. Meal: Vegan chickpea salad

2. Snack: Greek yogurt

3. Meal: Cauliflower rice and Teriyaki chicken

4. Snack: Glass of wine and cheese

Friday (Day 5)

1. Meal: Grilled salmon with mixed greens and brown rice

2. Snack: Pita and hummus with raw veggie sticks

3. Meal: Seared salmon with parmesan-kale salad and brown rice

4. Snack: Baked apple with cinnamon

Saturday (Day 6)

1. Meal: Avocado salad with chicken

2. Snack: Apricot slices with some mixed nuts

3. Meal: Pasta (Macadamia basil pesto)

4. Snack: Two chocolate chip cookies and a glass of milk

Sunday (Day 7)

1. Meal: Turkey chili with cornbread

2. Snack: Almond slices and Organic edamame

3. Meal: Asian fried noodles

4. Snack: Fruit salad

10.4 Intermittent Fasting Meal Plan for the Beginners

If you're new to fasting, begin by just eating between 8am. & 6pm. is the perfect way. This plan helps you consume all of your meals and snacks while still fasting for 14 hours in 24 hours.

1. Breakfast: Green Smoothie at 8 a.m.

Start the day of intake with smoothie after fasting because it is easier to digest for the gut. To stop a blood-sugar roller coaster, go for green smoothie rather than high-sugar fruit smoothie in the morning. To have you occupied until lunch, have plenty of the healthy fats.

Ingredients

- 1 small handful of blueberries
- 1 avocado
- one cup of coconut milk
- one tablespoon of chia seeds
- one cup kale, spinach, or chard

Instructions

Add all the ingredients together into a blender, mix, and enjoy!

2. Lunch: Grass-Fed Burgers at noon.

liver and Grass-fed burgers are 1 of the best weekday lunch options, and they're super easy to prepare ahead of time to enjoy during the week. It can be served over a layer of dark and leafy greens alongwith easy homemade dressings for B vitamin-rich meals that promote detox pathways and safe methylation.

Ingredients

- half tsp cumin powder
- half pound of grass-fed ground beef liver
- cooking oil as Desired
- half pound of grass-fed ground beef
- half teaspoon of garlic powder
- pepper and Sea salt to taste

Instructions

1. In a mixing bowl, combine all ingredients and shape into patties of desired size.
2. On a medium-high heat, heat the cooking oil in a skillet.
3. Cook the burgers in a skillet until done.
4. Refrigerate in an airtight container.

3. Snack: Cinnamon Roll Fat Bombs at 2:30 p.m.

The Fat bombs would satisfy the sweet tooth when providing sufficient healthy fat to have you going until dinner, & they taste just like cinnamon rolls.

Ingredients

- one tablespoon of coconut oil
- half cup of coconut cream
- one teaspoon cinnamon
- two tablespoons of almond butter

Instructions

1. Combine the coconut cream & half teaspoon cinnamon in a mixing bowl.
2. Cover the bottom of 8/8" four-sided pan with the parchment paper, then spread the cinnamon mixture and coconut cream.
3. Combine 1/2 teaspoon coconut oil, 1/2 teaspoon cinnamon, and 1/2 teaspoon almond butter. Then Spread over the pan's first layer.
4. Freeze for ten mins before cutting into squares or the bars.

4. Dinner: Salmon & Veggies at 5:30 p.m.

Dark green vegetables like broccoli and kale are rich in antioxidants, and salmon is an important source of omega-3 good fats. Salmon is important because of its taste & nutrient density, nonetheless you can use any wild-catch seafood you want. Serve with some of the favorite roasted vegetables in the coconut oil for a simple and quick super food meal.

Ingredients

- 2 tbsp ghee
- one pound of salmon or any other fish you like
- two tablespoons of lemon juice, fresh
- four finely diced cloves of garlic,

Instructions

1. Preheat the oven at 400 degrees Fahrenheit.
2. Combine the ghee, lemon juice, and garlic in a mixing bowl.
3. Place the salmon in the foil and cover with the lemon & ghee mixture.
4. Wrap the foil around the salmon and put it on the baking sheet.
5. Bake for fifteen mins or until the salmon is evenly cooked.
6. On another baking sheet, roast the vegetables alongside the salmon.

Conclusion

According to Luke Corey, a registered dietitian, intermittent fasting is a weight-loss strategy that first gained attention ten years ago. Intermittent fasting can boost indicators of mental and physical health and has an anti-aging impact. In addition to this it has also reported weight loss benefits.

Intermittent fasting is a catch-all word for a variety of fasting protocols. The basic idea is to eat food within a certain time frame. You eat very little to no food outside of that window.

Intermittent fasting advantages can be increased if you exercise regularly. Working out or exercising should be done at the end of the fasting window. It will help to get the most benefit. It's important to schedule the exercise to finish just as the eating window is about to begin.

It's critical to consult with a specialist in the area who has experience organizing these programs before beginning an intermittent fasting regimen. Those who do not properly set up the feeding windows with the right nutritional schedule risk losing muscle mass and not gaining the full benefits of implementing such a protocol.

Intermittent fasting is a healthy and reliable weight loss, anti-aging, and overall health strategy. It encourages people to think about the food they're eating and why they're eating it. It has the potential to be a beneficial plan for a large number of people.

9 781802 345360